Miracle Baby

Miracle Baby

A Fertility Doctor's Fight For Motherhood

Dorette Noorhasan, MD

BROWN BOOKS
PUBLISHING GROUP

Miracle Baby
A Fertility Doctor's Fight for Motherhood

Brown Books Publishing Group
16250 Knoll Trail Drive, Suite 205
Dallas, Texas 75248
www.BrownBooks.com
(972) 381-0009

A New Era in Publishing®

Publisher's Cataloging-In-Publication Data
Names: Noorhasan, Dorette, author.
Title: Miracle baby : a fertility doctor's fight for motherhood / Dorette
    Noorhasan, MD.
Description: Dallas, Texas : Brown Books Publishing Group, [2019]
Identifiers: ISBN 9781612543130
Subjects: LCSH: Noorhasan, Dorette. | Women gynecologists--United States-
    -Biography. | Infertility, Female--Patients--United States--Biography. |
    Motherhood. | LCGFT: Autobiographies.
Classification: LCC RG76.N66 A3 2019 | DDC 618.10092--dc23

ISBN 978-1-61254-313-0
LCCN 2019933944

Printed in the United States
10 9 8 7 6 5 4 3 2 1

For more information or to contact the author, please go to
www.DrDoretteNoorhasan.com.

This book is dedicated to all my positive influences: my parents, who were immigrants and made tremendous sacrifices for me to be where I am now; my maternal grandmother, who taught me to be the woman that I am today; my loving husband and best friend, who is my strongest supporter; my son, who brings me more joy than I could possibly describe in words—a joy that only another mother could understand; and my patients, who inspire me every day.

CONTENTS

One

The Delivery

She sat in the hospital bed, playing various games on her phone and conversing calmly with everyone in the room. Her epidural was working well—no one would ever guess that she was in active labor. This was her third pregnancy, her first as a surrogate. Although it had been a year since Kayla and I met, we were two strangers now sharing a very intimate moment. She was giving birth to my son—a child who was genetically related to me and my husband, Mike, but whom she had carried for nine months. At that point in time, she knew more about his habits than I did.

Kayla and I had met just a year ago through a surrogacy agency, but I couldn't believe how close we'd grown in that year. Although this was her first surrogacy journey, Kayla was very familiar with fertility treatments, since she had utilized in vitro fertilization (IVF) to have her three children (twins first, then a singleton). Kayla had two more frozen embryos but did not want five children, so in order to emotionally come full circle regarding not using her two remaining embryos, she decided that she would give birth to two more children that were not hers. Surrogacy was the way to accomplish her goal and, at the same time, help another couple fulfill their dreams of having children—a dream Kayla was all too familiar with. She and I were both type A and aligned on many concepts regarding pregnancy, so it was a match made in heaven. After interviewing twelve women, Mike and I had been worried that the right surrogate did not exist!

As a fertility physician, I have been asked numerous times how difficult it is to find a surrogate. It is very difficult. First of all, there are not a lot of women who want to be surrogates. Even though they are compensated, many do not want to willingly have their bodies go through pregnancy and delivery without getting a baby to take home. Also, the surrogate's partner and family must make many personal sacrifices. Children might not understand that even though their mother is pregnant, there will not be a sibling to add to the family. And even finding the right surrogate on paper does not mean that the intended parent will have an emotional connection with the surrogate. Surrogacy is such an intimate choice that being united on the same decision-making process during the pregnancy is a must to avoid surprises down the road.

The night before our son's birth, we arrived in the small town of Kyle, Texas, where we checked into a local hotel. My husband, Mike, and I opened a bottle of champagne that night; we were toasting both to becoming parents and to our last night together without having to hire a babysitter. We woke up at 4:30 a.m. on delivery day in order to pick up Kayla at her house and arrive at the hospital for a 6:00 a.m. admission. We were all anxious. Although I am a well-accomplished physician who has delivered just under a thousand babies during my four-year residency program—and who, as a fertility doctor, has helped thousands more people conceive—I was nervous about taking on the new role of a mother who would be responsible for a child. On delivery day, was I going to wear my doctor hat or my mother hat? Throughout this entire process, I had done a decent job of separating fact from emotion. Kayla's obstetrician had offered me the opportunity to "catch" the baby upon delivery, but I told him that on this special day, I wanted to be only a mother.

That car ride to the hospital was unbelievably quiet. We were all still trying to wake up, and we were tense, not knowing what to expect that day. Even though my medical knowledge had been more of a help than a hindrance during this process, sometimes knowing too much can hurt you. I was worried that something would go wrong at delivery, and I was so habituated to disappointment that the thought of my dream coming true—of becoming a mother—scared me. I desperately wanted everything to work out fine with the delivery. I kept thinking that Kayla might not go into labor and would require a cesarean section or that there might be complications. What if the baby didn't survive? I did not know my son at that time, yet he was capable of eliciting all sorts of emotions in me.

After we registered at hospital admissions, Mike and I went to have breakfast while Kayla checked into the labor, delivery, and recovery (LDR) room. Kayla got situated in the room and had her epidural; she was already three centimeters dilated at admission. The doctor broke her bag of water, and she quickly progressed to five centimeters. Kayla advanced through labor easily on Pitocin, a medicine used to augment labor. Her fetal and labor monitoring strips were perfect, and in just a few hours, she was ten centimeters dilated. At lunchtime, the hospital staff started the preparations for delivery. They brought in the delivery tray, containing all the necessary instruments. Mike, who knows nothing about medical care, looked at the delivery tray and almost passed out—blood draws, medical procedures, and hospitals make him queasy. The pediatric nurse came into the LDR room and prepared the newborn area, which included connecting a suction device to the wall so that mucus and meconium (fetal poop) could be removed from the baby's airway at delivery. The noise of the wall suction made my husband even more nervous. The obstetrician arrived; Kayla started pushing; and after only five minutes, the baby was out. Kayla made everything look so simple. Mike and I, grateful that everything had gone so well, were both excited and nervous to meet our son. We had joked earlier that morning that even if he were an ugly baby, we would still love him. The doctor gave Mike scissors to cut the umbilical cord, but his hands were shaking so much that I doubted he would succeed. Medical equipment always elicits a vasovagal response in Mike, affecting his heart rate; he even has to lie down just to get his blood drawn. Though he was a kind man who'd donated blood in the past, the blood bank had told him not to return since he passed out the last time he was there.

To my surprise, Mike did a good job cutting the umbilical cord, after which the doctor passed the baby off to the pediatric nurse. We followed and watched as they cleaned the baby. Mike's immediate comment was that our son looked like my dad; even though his face was swollen, his eyes shut, and his skin covered in bodily fluids, we were able to decipher whom he looked like. Over the next months, our son would change his facial expression to look like various relatives on both sides of the family. Our son was cooperative with the nurse, crying quickly and demonstrating the signs that she was looking for. Thankfully, he had ten fingers and ten toes. I sighed with relief because he seemed OK.

My only request that day was that, after the baby was cleaned up, I wanted to be the first person to hold him. The nurse washed him, swaddled him, and handed him to me. I had held many babies in the past; in fact, I had been eleven years old when my parents had my brother and I became responsible for some of my brother's care. In addition, I had hugged countless babies whose parents I had assisted in conceiving. But until this point, I had never held a baby that was *mine*. My son captivated me the first time I held him, and I started crying even more than he had that day. I tried so hard to hold back the tears, as I am generally not a person of many emotions. Because of the many things I've endured in my personal life and seen in my professional life, I am excellent at hiding emotions, but I could not suppress the abundance of tears rolling down my cheeks. Very soon, I had a small river below my feet, and everyone in the delivery room was looking at me. I felt eyes piercing through my body, but I only wanted to look at my son. One of the nurses started to cry as well; I guess it is true that tears of joy are contagious.

During my first cuddle time with my son, I started talking to him. He looked me in the eye, as if he knew who I was even though I was not the one who had carried him for nine months. He had never smelled me or heard my voice; yet, somehow, I felt connected to him. Earlier that day, I had told my husband that I would hold the baby for just a few seconds, then pass our child to him. But I could not let go of our son; I just kept staring at him. In my eyes, he was everything that this mother could want.

Finally, I gave my husband the opportunity to hold our son. Although the nurses had asked me earlier whether I wanted to have skin-to-skin contact with the baby, I was too embarrassed to do so in the LDR room. Mike, however, was thrilled to have his turn, quickly lifting his sweater and bringing our son to his chest. The joy of watching the excitement on my husband's face brought even more tears to my eyes.

We named our son Leo. Except for Mike and me, no one had known his name. The previous year, before we met Kayla and started this process, we had hiked in Hot Springs, Arkansas. My husband gives pet names to the geckos in our yard, and he informed me during that hike that if we ever had a son, he wanted to name him Leopold after the new gecko he had noticed. Well, I was not exactly passionate about *Leopold*, but I did like *Leo*. It could be short for Leopold (which would make my husband happy) or for Leonardo (which would make my nephews happy, as they were avid *Teenage Mutant Ninja Turtle* fans), and it was the first three initials of my dad's name (which would make my dad happy). Hence, all the men in my life would be thrilled with that name. Hopefully, my son will be happy about it someday too.

Two

Where It All Started

I was born in Guyana, the only English-speaking country in South America. Many times, when I tell people I was born in Guyana, they immediately confuse it with Ghana in Africa. There were originally three Guianas in South America—British, French, and Dutch. British Guiana was a colony of Britain until 1966, when it attained its independence and was renamed Guyana. My parents, who were born when it was British Guiana and were there for Guyana's independence, still have many British customs. For example, they still call a quarter a shilling, and they spell words like "neighbor" and "labor" as "neighbour" and "labour." They also celebrate Boxing Day on December 26. I clearly remember my parents using the word "porridge" to describe hot oatmeal, cream of wheat, or any type of cereal or grain boiled in hot water or milk—a very British thing to do.

I have very few memories of Guyana, but great ones: our home, the nursery school that I attended, and my enthusiasm for dance. I remember winning a book as part of a dance competition in nursery school—dancing and having more books to read being two of my favorite things. I recall a fun experience in nursery school, in which I was struggling with writing the small letter *r*. One of my classmates felt sorry for me and helped me to write it. We had good neighbors in Guyana, where everyone treated each other like family. Our neighbors had two older boys who were like my big brothers and who would walk with me to school and back home every day. I reconnected with them several years ago in New York, where they now live. When I met them there, they welcomed me with open arms and remembered taking care of me.

My parents had three children in Guyana, including myself, the firstborn. The next daughter, Marie, was born fourteen months after me, and the third, Tashe, when I was about two and a half years old. I remember Tashe's birth—probably my first memory. At that time, children were not allowed in the hospital, so I could not visit Mom and Tashe inside. One of my dad's friends, who was like an uncle to me, brought me to the hospital's parking lot, and my mom stood at the window with the baby so I could see her.

Throughout my childhood, my parents told me lots of stories about their upbringing in Guyana. Dad was the oldest of seven children, though one died at a very young age, so I only knew of five of his siblings. My dad's mom was Indian, and his dad was Chinese. In photos of my grandfather and my dad, it was clear that my dad resembled the Indian side of the family, whereas my grandfather, on the other hand, was a classic Chinese-looking man who tied his long hair in a bun on top of his head, very much like the guys I saw in kung fu movies as a child. My grandfather died when I was a child, so I have very few memories of him. He was the town's dispenser—sort of like a modern-day pharmacist—and he was brilliant in the sciences. He told me stories about red and white blood cells; I remember him saying that red cells were good for blood and white cells helped fight off infections.

Grandfather passed on his wits to my dad, who is also a brilliant man. Unfortunately, his family grew up very poor; my dad had only two outfits at a time. He had to wash one by hand to be ready to wear it in a couple of days, and he did not own underwear until his teen years. His family did not have electricity or modern-day plumbing. My dad studied by candlelight at night and used the outhouse as a bathroom. Since he did not have a shower, he had to use a bucket of water for bathing. Although they were a large, poor family, they were happy. Dad excelled academically, finishing the equivalent of high school with advanced placement in every subject. As the oldest of six children, he went into the workforce straight out of high school to help support his family.

My maternal grandmother, "Granny," was the most influential person in my life—she taught me to be the woman that I am today. She assured me that education was the secret to success. Granny was born into a very wealthy Indian family in Guyana. Her biological mother, like Granny herself, was incredibly beautiful and ridiculously smart. A distant cousin recently described to me how his heart melted the first time he saw Granny, for Granny captured the eyes of many men. Granny was born out of wedlock and hence was a neglected baby. An elder woman visiting her home at that time noticed the neglected child who had essentially been left to die. She was able to get the child adopted by Queene, the only mother that Granny knew. Although they lived a very simple life, like my dad, my grandmother described a fulfilling childhood. In the 1930s, in a developing country, female children attended only elementary school; then they had to learn how to do chores around the house, cook, and find a good husband. This irritated Granny quite a bit, and it was not what she wanted. Since Granny was the one who taught me the importance of an education, she would have been proud to know that today, all three of her granddaughters have doctorate degrees.

Besides instilling in me the importance of an education, Granny explained the reality of life, something that a young child could not naturally understand. She taught me that God and the Church were the way of life, so I went to Church every Sunday—not because she told me that that was the right thing to do but because I wanted to go. I realized how smart I was and studied to earn an A on every test. It was clear that I could better myself through education, but it is a shame that Granny did not have the same opportunity to further her education beyond elementary school, as she was brilliant. Although she had severe insulin-dependent diabetes—a disease that she ultimately succumbed to—it was her drive and determination that was infectious.

Granny dated my maternal grandfather briefly, but the relationship did not last; however, they had a child, my mother. My grandfather was a greedy, deceitful lawyer in town, but that did not stop Granny from doing a fantastic job raising my mother. Queene and the extended adoptive family helped her out while Granny kept a very steady job as a telephone operator in town. She was liked extraordinarily well by her coworkers and everyone she encountered. According to my mom, Granny had many more suitors, but she was tired of empty promises. Granny was an independent, modern-day working woman trapped in a third-world country in the 1940s and '50s.

My mom—Dorette, for whom I was named—was an only child. She grew up with Queene's extended family and was showered with more love than she could ever imagine. Electricity was on and off very frequently, but her family had a fridge, unlike many others in their neighborhood. However, because power was an uncertainty, they never bought a lot of groceries to keep in the fridge; they went to the local butcher when they needed fresh meat to cook and purchased fresh milk from a nearby farmer when they needed dairy. Cooking was done with a gas stove, as electric stoves were not common there, and gas stoves were more reliable. The family did have a toilet and a shower in the house, but without reliable electricity to pump water upstairs, they often lifted a bucket of water upstairs for flushing. Also, my mom took great pride in having well-ironed clothes, which required a piece of heavy iron metal with a flat side that they put on the stove top. Once this piece of iron was hot, they picked it up with a pot holder and used it to iron their clothes.

My mother worked for an insurance agency. Every Friday afternoon, she took the insurance money to the nearby bank for deposit, where my dad worked as a teller. My dad says he fell in love with my mom the first time he saw her. He learned her schedule and made himself available every Friday to be her teller, which quickly led to a romance. They were married in a beautiful ceremony. Queene's daughter, Aunt Hyacinth, did an amazing job with my mom's hair and makeup, and she looked extraordinarily beautiful on her wedding day.

When they got married, my parents were young, in their early twenties, so they did not have a dime to their names. Granny bought a plot of land and gave it to my parents to build a home, which they were so proud of. Many relatives came by to visit. Even though we left Guyana when I was four years old, I have an abundance of lively memories of that house.

I was born three years after my parents' marriage. Prenatal care was not good in a developing country in the 1970s; it is probably not any better in these countries today. Although she might have occasionally seen a doctor during the pregnancy, I doubt my mother had adequate prenatal care—not because she was noncompliant but because prenatal care was not readily accessible.

My mom did not know whether she was having a boy or girl, but since her periods were normal, she did have some idea of her expected date of delivery. Unfortunately, she had a very traumatic delivery with me. Now, as a physician and mother, I can only imagine what she went through. Mom was a young woman brought up in a loving—maybe even somewhat sheltered—environment. Although she was petite, weighing only ninety-eight pounds, her belly was enormous. There were no ultrasounds available, so, for a long time, she thought she was having twins. The stretch marks on her belly were tortuous; she often described them as "snakelike."

Mom eventually went into labor well after her due date and was in labor for days; she thought I was not going to come out. I was delivered by forceps and still have a scar on my forehead from the delivery. My mom always told me that I was too comfortable in her uterus and did not want to leave. She said that her body never felt the same after her first pregnancy and delivery. As a physician and mother, I now know that, many times, the first pregnancy is difficult, and this experience certainly is worse in areas of the world where there is a lack of adequate medical care.

At the end of the 1970s, the political environment in Guyana became very unstable—and, sadly, is still the same or maybe even worse today. Guyana is a country unbelievably rich in natural resources, yet its people still suffer. We were lucky, as my dad received a promotion right around that time, and the company transferred him and our family to Belize.

Three

My First Experience with Death

In Belize, my family lived near the water, and it was very nice to go for a walk along the boardwalk near our home. Since I was the oldest of three daughters, I already had the "eldest sibling attributes." I quickly became involved with taking care of my younger siblings, as my mom was pregnant with her fourth child while we were living there. I was elated. Interestingly, infertility was not a problem in our family; my parents eventually had six children, four of whom are alive today. Mom had a traumatic delivery with me, but she had a much easier experience with my siblings, including this fourth pregnancy.

The fourth child was another girl, and she was the most precious baby I had ever seen. Her name was Lendorita—a combination of my parents' names and mine. Middle names were often used in our family—in fact, I did not know what my first name was until grade school, since my parents called me Juanie, an abbreviation of my middle name, Juanita. Like all of us siblings, my new sister was called by an abbreviation of her middle name: Nikki, short for Nicolasas.

As the youngest of four siblings, Nikki was so extraordinarily loved, and we all doted on her. My other sisters and I would fight over who got to hold Nikki or feed her. Our entire family revolved around this baby, who had incredibly fair skin, a full head of curly, jet-black hair, and giant brown "puppy-dog eyes."

However, at seven months of age, Nikki developed severe vomiting and diarrhea. She could not keep anything down, and she was lethargic. Since Mom did not know how to drive, she called Dad to pick her up on his lunch break to take her and Nikki to the hospital. On the drive there, Nikki passed away. My mom told my dad during the drive, "I think the baby just died in my arms." She has always told me that the worst death she has experienced was the death of child she had grown to know and love, which was worse than losing a parent. Now that I am a parent, I can only imagine what my mother went through. Nikki died of a gastrointestinal bug, which I now know is something easily treatable in many cases. I saw the tiny casket descend six feet into the ground. A few days later, I went to Nikki's bed and started to cry. No, I was bawling. I was then five years old and understood death; I knew that I was not going to see Nikki ever again. Nikki's death planted a seed in me to pursue medicine. At the age of just five, it broke my heart to see women and children suffer.

I started kindergarten a few months later. I was elated to meet more kids and friends because before that in Belize, I had only been exposed to my siblings. While growing up with siblings means you always have playmates, it was different for me. Having younger siblings meant that I had to take care of them and keep them out of trouble, so it was exciting to make friends that I could just play with without having to assume caregiving responsibilities. I attended St. Joseph's elementary school in Belize, which, in the eyes of a five-year-old, was a large school. There were big kids there—sixth graders, that is. I really wanted to hang out with the older kids because they seemed to have so much fun, but I was stuck in a tiny five-year-old body. I quickly made many friends among kids my age, and I always had a group to have lunch with and to play with during recess breaks. In our schoolyard were several maypoles—vertical poles that we danced around, wrapping various ribbon designs during school festivities. This was one of my favorite things to do. It was celebratory to listen to music and dance in circular designs around the pole, resulting in a pole wrapped in a beautiful ribbon pattern.

While living in Belize, our family bought our first television—a small, thirteen-inch, black-and-white box. We were so proud to have a TV; it was a privilege. I loved music, and Michael Jackson was a big deal back then. His "Thriller," "Beat It," and "Pretty Young Thing" were among my favorites. One of the kids in our neighborhood and I had developed a complete dance routine for "Beat It." Our parents loved it, and pretty soon, we had my younger siblings doing the routine. Dancing was such a good pastime; we would stop and dance whenever we passed by musicians playing in the streets. So, my sisters and I quickly became little entertainers.

We lived in Belize until I was about seven years old, when my father was transferred, with the company, to Antigua. I was sad once again to leave my friends and have to go to a new place, learn my way around, attend a new school, and make new friends. But there was the adventurous part of me that was excited to go live in another location of the world and learn about that environment. So, my family packed up and moved to Antigua.

Four

A Happy Childhood

We arrived in Antigua just in time for Christmas, the school break being a good time for a move. My sisters and I could end the old semester in Belize and start the new one in Antigua. It was an exciting time for my jovial family—we love to celebrate all holidays, Christmas being the most celebratory. This was a special Christmas because we were starting a new life in Antigua. Since my sisters and I were unbelievably curious kids, we already knew that Santa was not real and that our parents bought the gifts and placed them under the Christmas tree the night before. That year, while unpacking, we came across a large bag filled with gifts—three of everything, just in different colors, to perfectly match three girls. We were sure we had found the loot, but instead of pretending that we had not found the gifts, we confessed. However, it turned out that we still had to wait until Christmas to receive them!

It took us some time to assimilate to Antiguan culture. While we are Episcopalian (Anglican, in the English system), we attended Holy Family Elementary School, a Catholic school, because our parents wanted us to go to a good Christian school. Holy Family Elementary was stricter than the other schools I had attended. Nuns ran the school system. Although they were gentle and kind, they were very disciplined and expected similar behavior from all the students. We addressed the nuns by calling them "Sister" followed by their first names. Most of the kids who attended the school, like myself, did not get into trouble; after all, only kids whose parents thought they would fit in the school attended. Even though I did not know anyone who was expelled, I was sure it would happen if any child seriously misbehaved. We stood at attention every morning for the singing of Antigua's national anthem, and every Wednesday, we had Mass in the chapel. Going to the chapel meant singing cool hymns.

Another reason it took my sisters and I some time to assimilate with the other kids was that we were starting school in the middle of the school year. Additionally, we were not from Antigua, and some of the other kids were fascinated to see kids of Asian descent. The population there was mostly black, with a minority of white children; we were the only Asian kids in the school at that time. My sister Marie, who was born fourteen months after me, was almost as tall as I was, so everyone thought we were twins, which made us even more interesting. While Marie was quiet and shy, I quickly became buddies with everyone and got to participate in the popular games. There were no cliques there; everyone was friendly and welcoming. So as long as we took initiative to get to know the other students, we quickly made friends.

We played lots of fun games in the schoolyard at recess, so I came home numerous times with bruises and cuts from playing "catch." Most of these were minor; I remember just two large cuts. I have a large scar on my right elbow from a big accident, and both of my knees have many scars from falls. However, I did even more damage to myself at home. One day, I wore my mom's heels around the house, because, like any girl, I considered it "cute." But the shoes were too big for me, and I slipped and fell down the stairs, striking my back on each step. On another occasion, I broke my nose after swinging off the chairs in the living room and falling face first into the concrete floor. As a result, I had massive bleeding from my nose for a few hours, with severe pain and sporadic bleeding for several weeks. This—in addition to my allergies—is probably why I have had some breathing issues as an adult, but at least it was a fun childhood.

While we were in elementary school, my sister and I joined the Brownies, which was a great way for us to meet more friends our age. We quickly became involved in several activities, including field trips that allowed us to hike small hills and learn about the wildlife around us. We did volunteer work, such as cleaning the schoolyard after school once per month, and we felt a strong sense of accomplishment earning badges.

Holy Family merged with another Catholic school, Christ the King, just before I started the fourth grade. Because the school was now bigger, the church was able to save money to build a large, beautiful cathedral for the students to attend services in. I was very happy then; I had lots of friends and enjoyed every day of my life at school. We also had many friends in our neighborhood, so I had kids to play with after school. One of the neighbors who lived four streets over started a weekly Bible study after school, and we all had so much fun going over various stories in the Bible. Additionally, we participated in weekend camping trips, where I learned how to make s'mores and a few other over-the-fire quick eats. However, I was still too young to try to start the fire for the camping trips; only the adults were allowed to do that.

In our family, we were trained to address all adults as "Auntie" or "Uncle" even if they were not related to us, and we were not allowed to call any adult by only their first name. Auntie Mae and Uncle Michael lived across from us. Uncle Michael was a carpenter—more like a modern-day contractor—who had built their home essentially with his bare hands. It was one of the most beautiful homes I had ever seen at that time. Auntie Mae was skilled at decorating—walking through their home was like walking through a showroom, an immaculate model house. She was also good at baking, and I loved going over to their house for freshly baked cookies. Unfortunately, later in life, Auntie Mae struggled with diabetes, which she eventually succumbed to. Auntie Mae and Uncle Michael were the most perfect couple, living a love story that most women can only fantasize about. Uncle Michael always looked at Auntie Mae with so much love in his eyes. And why not? She was an amazing woman, and their love was infectious. They had a daughter, Amanda, who was maybe only four years older than me. But she had already undergone puberty, and I was just a scrawny kid. Amanda carpooled with us to school since, after the school merger, the high school was now on the same campus as the elementary school. I really enjoyed interacting with her on the car rides; she was like the older sister that I never had.

Auntie Margaret lived two doors over. She was my new godmother since my old godmother in Guyana was not with us. I had completed all my Bible studies at the church we attended and was ready for my confirmation and First Communion. I was elated—this was a big step for me. As a gift, Auntie Margaret bought me a Bible that still sits on my nightstand to this day. I was like a daughter to Auntie Margaret, who struggled with infertility. In the meantime, she spoiled me with all the love that she wanted to give to a daughter, and I absolutely enjoyed all her attention. This was my first exposure to infertility, though at nine years old, I did not understand the details. I heard Auntie Margaret and my mom talking about her struggles with having a baby; Auntie Margaret was in tears. I felt terrible for her because she was such a nice woman who showed me unconditional love. When I was growing up, I went over to her house several times after school to keep her company, and in many ways, I became her adopted daughter. I wished that she could also have a daughter—and, indeed, my wish eventually came true. Right around the time we moved from Antigua, I heard that Auntie Margaret was expecting a little girl!

Auntie Rosa and Uncle Matt were our neighbors immediately next door. They had a daughter, Marie, who was about two years younger than me—more my sisters' ages, not mine. Besides, I liked playing with older kids. One school day while Uncle Matt and Marie were at work and school, respectively, an intruder walked in on Auntie Rosa through a door she had left open. The intruder stole many items while she was asleep in the living room chair, but she was lucky that he caused her no harm. Since we lived right next door to them, that could easily have happened to my mom while I was in school. We were lucky that the intruder did not target us. Auntie Rosa and Uncle Matt always kissed in front of everyone and appeared to be a loving couple, although certainly not the genuine love I saw with Auntie Mae and Uncle Michael. Later, I found out that Auntie Rosa and Uncle Matt divorced a few years after we left Antigua.

In Antigua, I quickly became involved in our church, where I attended Bible school and volunteered for many church-related activities. There were just two problems. Firstly, neither I nor my mother could drive. So, I relied on my dad to shuttle me to all the events that did not affect his work schedule. Furthermore, I had some clothes but did not have a lot of nice church dresses to keep up with the other girls. Since we wore uniforms for school, my parents did not spend money buying street clothes and church clothes. My mom had an interest in arts, crafts, and sewing, and Auntie Mae was a great influence on her. Auntie taught my mom how to shop for material and patterns and how to sew cute clothes for me to go to church events. I quickly went from a sparse closet to having no room to add more clothes. Mom was on a sewing high; the more she sewed, the more confident she became to sew more complicated dresses the next time. Later in life, my mom sewed my prom dress and some very complex evening gowns for me. She was a good influence on my sisters and me—we now sewed for our Barbie dolls. Every summer, we had "Miss Barbie of the World" competitions, in which my sisters and I sewed evening gowns for our dolls and had them model for our parents. Our parents were the judges, selecting the best-dressed Barbie, who got to wear an aluminum foil crown.

Five

A Very Sad Eighth Birthday

My mom conceived again for the fifth time, pregnant with another girl. Granny now lived with us in Antigua, so she was instrumental in helping my mom, who was juggling three children and house chores. On top of that, we did not have a microwave, washing machine, or dishwasher. Granny and Mom made a new meal three times per day from scratch, and they used a washing board to scrub our clothes clean before hanging them in the sunlight to dry. During her pregnancy, my dad convinced my mother to go stay with his relatives in St. Croix, as it was a United States territory, and he thought she would get better medical care there. My parents were still traumatized by Nikki's death. Dad's siblings had left Guyana and moved to St. Croix right around the time we moved to Belize, so my mom spent her last trimester in St. Croix, staying with her in-laws while Granny took care of us three girls at home in Antigua.

In St. Croix, my mother went for all her prenatal appointments, and everything seemed to be going well. She went into labor on my eighth birthday, but when she showed up to the hospital, the baby no longer had a fetal heart beat, even though it had had a heart beat the week before. So, on my eighth birthday—what should have been a happy day for me—I learned not only that my younger sister had been born that day but that she had not lived and I would never meet her. I was told that my sister, Andromeda, had been incredibly beautiful. She was named after Andromeda in Greek mythology; however, the Andromeda in Greek mythology was saved by Perseus. No one saved my sister.

Since then, I have never celebrated another birthday. *If one of us was going to die*, I wondered, *why the baby? Why was I saved?* It is hard to celebrate my birthday when Andromeda could not celebrate hers. It was my sister's stillbirth that stimulated my interest in obstetrics/gynecology. I wanted to know whether her death was due to my mom's prenatal care or could have been prevented. My desire was to learn how I could prevent this from happening to others. Then, I was too young to understand. Maybe now that I am educated about the process, I might be able to read my mom's medical records and learn exactly what happened. However, most hospitals are not required to keep records after a certain amount of years—usually somewhere between seven to ten, depending on state laws and hospital policies.

After losing two children consecutively, my mom was an emotional wreck. She and my dad had numerous fights regarding what they could have done differently, and the blame game continued for many months. A few years later—now pushing age forty—my mom conceived a sixth time. She was unbelievably scared and wished that she had never conceived again. She'd thought she was too old to have children. Apparently not. My parents fought a lot during this pregnancy. She wanted to stay in Antigua, where she was happy, but he wanted to move to St. Croix. In the end, she won this battle. Fortunately, Mom had excellent prenatal care with a doctor in Antigua. One day close to her delivery date, she came home from her prenatal appointment in tears. I clearly remember seeing my mother crying, because she rarely cried around us. She always tried to show a "strong" personality around her children. That day, however, she was afraid she was going to lose another child. Sadly, she now had severe preeclampsia—a condition in which a pregnant woman develops high blood pressure and loss of protein in her urine. With good medical care, many women do well. However, preeclampsia can lead to maternal seizures, fluid in the lungs of the mom, impaired maternal kidney and liver function, and, in rare cases, maternal and fetal deaths. My mom's blood pressure was through the roof, and her legs were larger than those of an elephant.

The doctor told her, "You need to deliver today, or there could be severe consequences, including losing the infant." Mom had lost her last two children and now was feeling impending doom that she would lose this one too. To make matters worse, this was her first boy. Therefore, she signed the consent form to have a cesarean section and her tubes tied—she did not want another pregnancy after this one. Thankfully, her delivery went smoothly. She received such good care in the hospital that all her anxiety vanished. My sisters and I were elated to have a brother, Shane. Needless to say, Shane is spoiled rotten since he is the youngest and only boy.

I was eleven years old around the time of Shane's birth, so, in many ways, I was his second mother. My mom leaned on me for help many times since I had a natural maternal instinct even though I was not ready to be a mother myself at that time. One of my mom's friends, Auntie Olivia, worked in a bar, and we always stopped by to see her on our way to the amusement park down the road. One evening, we headed back from the amusement park and stopped by the bar as usual. Auntie Olivia had made a batch of goat water (goat soup) and kept it in the fridge to give to my mom, so Mom followed her into the kitchen, asking me to hold Shane until she returned. My dad always bought a beer in the bar to support Auntie Olivia, and he decided that he needed to use the restroom before we drove home. He handed his unfinished beer to me to hold while he went to the restroom. A few minutes later, a woman walked into the bar. Even though I was eleven, I had full female characteristics and could have easily been mistaken for fourteen years old. The woman walked over to me and, in a very concerned voice, inquired why a teenage mother with her baby was in a bar holding a beer. I quickly told the woman that the baby was my brother and that I was holding my dad's beer until he returned from the restroom. I guess my maternal persona has always been a part of my identity.

After Shane's birth, my dad was now determined to move closer to his family in St. Croix, so his brother helped him and our family obtain our green cards so that we were able to move. My dad gave up a fantastic job that moved us all over the Caribbean to take a mediocre job in St. Croix, but we were moving to an American territory and closer to his family. I was always excited about a new adventure, even though I had an excellent school life in Antigua—a life that I had to put behind me and start all over once more.

Six

First Experiences in the US Virgin Islands

We had been going back and forth to St. Croix for a few years to visit my dad's family, but my mom insisted that if we were going to move to the US Virgin Islands, we should move to St. Thomas, not St. Croix. The death of Mom's fifth child had left her devastated. Although we had been in private school in Antigua, for financial reasons my parents decided to try the public school system in St. Thomas. We moved to St. Thomas in January of 1988; however, for whatever reason, it was three months before we could enroll in a school. By the time I got back to school, I had only three months before my sixth-grade graduation. The school environment was very different from what I had been familiar with in Antigua: the children were rude and disrespectful of adults, and they did not take their studies seriously. A boy had a crush on me, but I was certainly not interested, so one day he decided to show me his pecker to convince me that he was "all that." This only confirmed my lack of interest!

In school, my sisters and I stayed close together. We were very uncomfortable in the new school environment. We tried to find each other during the lunch break—this was in the days before cell phones. In Antigua, I'd had to pack my lunch the night before classes, but at this school, they gave free lunches. I absolutely enjoyed the chocolate milk they gave us at lunchtime; it was a new experience to get a lunch tray, stand in line, and tell the ladies behind the counter what I wanted to eat. I no longer needed my pirate-themed lunch box that I had used for so many years. Luckily, I graduated from the sixth grade and thus finished elementary school without a problem.

When I started seventh grade in the fall of 1988, my parents decided to put me in private school. Things were not as easy as when we lived in Antigua because my dad's income was not enough to make ends meet. Mom, who had not worked in at least twelve years, went back to work as an administrative assistant for a furniture company. Fortunately, Granny was with us to help. My brother, Shane, was only a year old, but Granny did an amazing job as an older woman taking care of an infant while doing all the housework and making our meals. We stayed in St. Thomas for only a year, after which Dad insisted we move to St. Croix so he could be closer to family. So, we moved to St. Croix during Christmas break in 1988.

We arrived in St. Croix in December 1988, and I took an exam at St. Dunstan's Episcopal School in January 1989. I was halfway through the seventh grade at that time, but I placed at an eighth-grade level on the entrance exam. After the vice principal made a comment to my mother regarding my score on the exam, Mom insisted that I be placed in the eighth grade since I could do the work. I had always been the smallest and youngest kid in the class, as I had started school one year early, but now that my mom had made me move up a grade, I now was two years younger than the kids sitting right next to me. At this school, the kids in my class were incredibly rude. When we'd lived in Antigua, I'd wanted to grow up to be a schoolteacher: I'd had so many excellent teachers influence my life, and I wanted to do the same for other children. Now, I changed my mind—there was no way I was going to be a schoolteacher to these rude, ungrateful kids! They hated me without even trying to get to know me.

My name is "Dorette," but my rude classmates had heard how smart I was and decided to call me "Nerdette." This was certainly a different experience than when I'd started school midyear in Antigua. I arrived home from my second day at school in tears, both sad and mad at my mom for making me be in a class with disrespectful older kids. Intellectually, I felt that I had not lived long enough or had the experience they did to spar with them over words. Granny saw me crying and said to me, "Twenty years from now, you will be the one laughing. They have peaked now, but you will peak at a later, more appropriate time." She reminded me how extraordinarily talented I was and that I should never let anyone put me down. Well, that was all I needed to hear. From that moment on, whenever I was teased in school, I just looked the other way and never responded. I already knew what my future looked like, but they did not know theirs. Six months later, I completed the eighth grade and was able to graduate from middle school. After only six months, I had the highest GPA of all the kids in the class, many of whom were almost two years older than me. Unfortunately, I had not attended the school long enough to qualify for the valedictorian spot in my graduating class, but I marched in the graduation and gratefully accepted my certificate anyway!

Granny taught me many good mottos for life, many of which I still live by. She could have lost her life as a baby, but she fought for everything she ever achieved. We were a Christian family that attended church every Sunday, and we lived our lives the way we believed God wanted us to. I prayed every night before I went to sleep; every morning when I rose from bed, I thanked God that I'd lived to see another sunrise, because some people, including my grandfather Carl, do not rise the next morning. I also prayed before each meal, thanking God that I had something to eat, since I had seen too many television commercials asking for money for children in Africa who were literally starving to death. One of the most important mottos Granny taught me was "God helps those who help themselves." Like many other children, I prayed to God to give me things, but Granny always reminded me that if I wanted something to happen in my life, I needed to get up and go after it, not sit down feeling sorry that it had not been given to me. So, I prayed for toys, but I also saved up my allowance so I could buy them. I then thanked God that my parents were healthy and worked to give me an allowance so I was able to buy the toys that I wanted. Another memorable motto Granny taught me was to always be grateful in life, because things could be much worse. This motto has helped me through countless situations. At times when I feel sad or that the world has been unfair to me, I start to count my blessings. Then I quickly see the cup as half full. This viewpoint has pulled me out of sad situations and quickly allowed me to see the bigger picture.

Every morning, Granny drank tea, a tradition that I still follow today. Tea was a big pastime in Guyana, most likely a tradition that had stayed since Guyana was once a British colony. One day, I came home after school to find that my younger sister Tashe had been playing in the dining room area and had accidentally pulled a cup of hot tea down onto herself. My family took her to the emergency room (ER) because she had severe burns along her right upper arm and the right side of her chest and was in so much pain. The hospital staff bandaged her up and told my parents how to take care of her. Although the burns eventually healed, they left large physical scars, which were probably not as bad as the emotional scars. Tashe was embarrassed to wear tank tops and always wore sleeves despite the hot climate. As a teenager, she was embarrassed in the girl's locker room since the burned area on her chest was now on her right breast. She is now a very well-adapted woman and mother, but I could only imagine what it took for her to get to a point in her life where she felt comfortable in her own body.

Seven

Hurricane Hugo

When we moved to St. Croix in December of 1988, we rented a small house not too far from the ocean. Even though rent was high, the house was in desperate need of repairs; nor was it set up in a functional way—for example, navigating from the dining room to the kitchen was next to impossible. Our parents no longer wanted to rent, so they decided to purchase a home, a small house catty corner to my Uncle Caesar's house in Clifton Hill, St. Croix. We moved in at the end of the summer of 1989, and I had just started the ninth grade when the island was hit by Hurricane Hugo. It was a terrifying hurricane. Although my parents had lived through some very large storms, they were nothing like Hurricane Hugo. Smartphones with fancy apps to track hurricanes were not available at that time, and the internet was in its infancy. We listened to the news on the television and the radio; the grocery stores distributed small maps on which we plotted the longitude and latitude of the hurricane to get an idea of Hugo's location. The news told us to stock up on nonperishable foods, toilet paper, and water and to board up our home, so we did. On September 17, 1989, the winds became stronger, and by the evening hours, the rain started. Power went out very early—it had been cut to avoid active electric wires coming down during the storm. Rain then came down heavier and heavier, practically relentless, and the wind was loud. We heard multiple crashing sounds as large trees fell over, some onto nearby cars (including ours, since we did not have a garage). Some of the trees had spiral bends to the trunks, suggestive of tornado-like wind damage. The back part of our house lost the roof; rain poured into the front part of the house, where we were residing. We used large blankets, old curtains, and towels to mop up as much of the water as possible, but more seeped in through the windows. Luckily, we had metal shutters rather than glass windows, yet still these could not stand up to the rain and wind. In the yard, we had a large breadfruit tree, which bore fruits similar in size to large coconuts; we heard each fruit hit the ground with a hard splatter. Then the tree was completely uprooted (despite its large, sturdy trunk) and thrown to another part of our yard. We were terrified for our lives.

Around 2:00 a.m., we heard a knock on our door. It was the neighbors across the street. My family and I were friendly and enjoyed getting acquainted with our neighbors, but since we had just moved in two weeks before, we had not had the chance to meet them. Their entire house had been ruined by the storm; they had been hiding in their bathroom until 2:00 a.m., at which point there was a calm as the eye of the hurricane passed. But the calm was deceiving—the eye of a hurricane only means that the next half is coming. So, our neighbors and their two children, ages five and two, ran out in the storm and knocked on our door, and we quickly brought them to shelter and gave them dry clothes. Some of my father's siblings and their families had also come over earlier that day to ride out the storm since they did not live in sturdy homes. By the end of the storm—and for the next three months—there were seventeen people living in the undamaged part of our home, which comprised about twelve hundred square feet of space. Clifton Hill is in the middle of the island on a small hill, so we were far away from the large tide surges on the coast. I could not imagine surviving having to deal with tide surges on top of the strong winds and rain. I guess that was why the government had told all residents living near the water that they had to evacuate that area.

The reality is that if you seek shelter ahead of time, you have a high chance of surviving a hurricane. The hardest part is the aftermath. By noon the next day, the weather was calming down, and there was just a sprinkle of rain. There were still strong winds, but nothing like what we had experienced the night before, so we came out to see what had happened. The island was truly annihilated, with debris everywhere. The cleanup took months. We started with the big debris and then slowly moved on to the smaller items. Even though we are a territory of the United States and, like all citizens, pay federal taxes, it took a long time before we saw any help. Homes that were still standing had blue tarps covering where roofs used to be, such as on the back part of our house. But we needed more than just a new roof—there had also been some structural damage when the roof came down. People were so desperate that, the day after the storm, we heard there was looting as people broke into homes and businesses.

To deal with the chaos, the government started a curfew at 6:00 p.m. There were lines for everything, including the grocery stores, which quickly sold out their old stock days before the next shipments would arrive. The grocery stores were powered by generators; luckily, we were able to buy a small generator for our home, though it only gave us about three to four hours of power at a time before we had to refill it with gas. But gas was in short supply, too, so there were lines at the gas station, and they limited how much gas each customer could buy to avoid some people buying out all the gas and leaving none for others. In addition to our fridge, we had a large freezer in the back of the house. Fortunately, my parents are the type of people who buy food in bulk and keep a full freezer, so we were able to eat the food out of our freezer over the next several days as the items slowly thawed out. We had a gas stove and had just bought a new tank of gas when we moved in, so we were able to cook. Once the freezer items were gone, we worked on the items in the pantry, and by the time our food supplies had run out, the grocery stores were full, and the Federal Emergency Management Agency (FEMA) and several other agencies had arrived with aid. I learned how to eat meals ready to eat (MREs), which were surprisingly, pleasantly edible. Some of the items just required reconstitution with water, and then we had full, ready-to-eat meals. It is amazing that certain food items do not taste bad when your choice is between eating them or not eating at all!

Water and power returned to government agencies, hospitals, and schools first. I returned to school just two weeks after the storm. Usually, we wore uniforms to school, but since some children had lost their entire homes (including their clothes), the school allowed us to wear street clothes for the rest of that school year. I was amazed at the resilience of the people of the Virgin Islands. We all went back to school and talked about the hurricane as if it had been just a small event. Although most of us did not have power in our homes and many of us were living with relatives until our homes could be rebuilt, it was back to learning as usual. Every day, I came home from school and did my homework before sundown, when we powered up the generator for a couple of hours so we could take baths, eat dinner, and get ready for bed. Life was a bit primitive, to say the least.

Without a doubt, though, Hurricane Hugo was a blessing for some of us. One of my classmates had been a swimmer until Hurricane Hugo hit. The hurricane ruined St. Croix's only Olympic-size swimming pool, so my classmate started playing basketball. You might know him as Tim Duncan, who became one of the superstars of the San Antonio Spurs. As Mom always said, "Everything happens for a reason." When one door closes, a better door is about to open.

Uncle Caesar was not so lucky. He lost his roof during Hurricane Hugo; additionally, there was a lot of water damage to the remainder of the house. You can imagine that if there is no roof, then nothing in the house is protected from the pouring rain and wind. We helped Uncle Caesar clean up the debris, and we rented a chain saw to cut down the tree branches hanging over his house and ours. He put up a tarp temporarily until he could get a new roof. Uncle Caesar was the cool uncle, single and a lot of fun, who took us out for ice cream and snow cones almost weekly.

Poor Uncle Caesar got really sick a few months after the hurricane. He had severe, bloody vomiting and was hospitalized for a long time. Though he recovered, he died twenty years later from esophageal cancer, as his esophagus had been ruined from the reflux of his gastric contents. When he was diagnosed with cancer, he was already stage IV, with immense weight loss, but he took his diagnosis calmly and went to New York City to be with extended relatives while he received medical care. However, it seemed that the medical treatment made him sicker. Uncle Caesar never lost his sense of humor, though, and he called me several times from the hospital in New York. I think he knew his time was coming. We had a close relationship, so he always wanted my opinion on his treatment. It was difficult for me to give him an opinion, though, because cancer is not my specialty and because—based on his symptoms and on him being stage IV—I knew that he had very little time left. Even still, I never told him that I thought his prognosis was poor, because I did not need to end his sense of hope and happiness with my realistic words. His treating physicians could do that; I was just a family member providing love and support to someone who really needed it. Uncle Caesar was a very pleasant, happy man until his last breath, for which I was grateful.

Power was restored to Clifton Hill almost three months following Hurricane Hugo. The saddest part of this was that we were not the last people to receive power, as it took many more months before the entire island recovered. That Christmas, we were extraordinarily grateful for power, life, love, and family. I do not even remember what Christmas gifts I received that year, for I had all that I wanted at that time; we had made it through a very difficult time in our lives.

Eight

My High School Life

After Hurricane Hugo, the rest of high school flew by. Academically, I continued to excel, but I now wanted to develop other talents. Dancing had always been an outlet for me; however, the reality was that I had not danced much since the second grade. I had been so engrossed in my studies that I'd forgotten about all the other things that excited me, and I was teased so much in school that I had lost all the self-esteem that I needed to pursue other things. On top of that, I was now wearing braces on my teeth and glasses. It could not get any worse.

In the tenth grade, I was able to take a dance class as an elective. The teacher was unbelievably talented and nice. She choreographed an amazing dance, which we performed at the local theater, and once that semester was over, I joined the local dance school in town, where she was a full-time instructor. Compared to some of the girls at the dance school, who had been dancing all their lives, I was very awkward at first. I signed up for classes in ballet, jazz, Afro-Caribbean, and modern dance. My parents were a bit old-school

Indian in their beliefs, so I was not able to convince them that I should do this, thus requiring that I save up the money to pay for my dance tuition. The dance school was just a five-minute drive from my dad's job, so I was able to coordinate with him to get a ride there. I loved dancing because it was so much fun, and in just a few months, I saw my body transform from skinny and nerdy to athletic and muscular. During this time, my grades never fell; if anything, they improved. I was now more efficient at getting my studies done so I could go to dance classes. After two years at the dance school, the owner of the school asked me to join the dance team and go on tour with them. Since I was about to graduate from high school and go to college, I knew that I would not be able to pour my heart into dancing and still transition into college, but the owner was determined. He went to my dad's job and asked his permission for me to join the dance team; my dad, however, insisted that his daughter made her own decisions. Dad never told me that story until about ten years later.

Because I am the oldest of my siblings, finding a summer job was financially helpful to my family. Plus, it gave me extra cash to pursue the things I wanted to do and taught me some basic money-management skills. In the ninth grade, I worked as a clerk in a bank, sitting in a small room with stacks of papers and old checks and looking for the right file cabinet to put them in. I did not have any interaction with anyone at the bank; it was just me in a filing room.

As soon as I learned the filing system, everything became easy. The next summer, I found a job at Kinney's shoe store as a cashier, a job I kept for the rest of high school and my first year in college. I was so good with a register and numbers that I quickly knew the totals well before the machine could tally things up. A lot of this came from my mom, whom I had watched do the shopping, during which she always made sure she stayed within her budget. The best part of my job at Kinney's was that it taught me more communication skills. Although I had been very friendly before this job, I now took the initiative to get to know my customers and make small talk, as I needed to make sales so I could earn my commission. I learned how to help people find the right shoes and try them on without turning up my nose at their stinky feet, and I also learned about shoe sizes and measurements. In addition, I got a nice discount, so I was able to buy Mom, Granny, and my sisters gifts from the store regularly. Pretty soon, my wardrobe had every shoe style in every color. Our uniforms at Kinney's included a tie, which my dad taught me how to tie. It felt so official wearing a tie to work.

I had to take a taxi van to and from my job at Kinney's; I could not wait to get my driver's license and gain some real independence. My parents are so old school that my mom had never learned to drive and had to rely on my dad for everything, but I was determined to be an independent woman and have a career. I asked—practically annoyed—my father until he taught me how to drive. Although he was not a patient teacher, I was determined that I would learn to drive. So, every Saturday morning, we got up and went for a drive around the island. I saw parts of the island that I had never seen before, discovering numerous back roads. I passed the written portion of my driver's test, but the first time I took the practical portion, I failed. The examiner for the practical portion was notorious for being incredibly difficult, and most students failed the driving test with him. When I learned that morning that he was going to accompany me in the car, I was a nervous wreck: I could not think straight because I was so afraid that he would yell at me. He did not yell. I was already doing such a good job intimidating myself that he did not have to do any of it. I was embarrassed when I failed, since I had excelled at everything but this one test. I questioned my plans to be an independent woman, especially since I needed to be able to get myself around in order to pursue my dreams. After a few days of feeling sorry for myself, I gave myself a pep talk and went ahead and registered to take the test again. My neighbor let me borrow her car to take the test, since on the first test, I'd used the car at the police station, which was big and bulky and had a stiff steering wheel. My neighbor's car, on the other hand, I had driven several times in the past; it was small and unbelievably easy to maneuver, and the steering wheel spun like melted butter on a frying pan. So, I was ready for my examining officer; he was no longer going to terrorize me. I walked in with my A game. Well, as luck would have it, I got a different examiner that day, a really nice police officer whose calming demeanor set my nerves at ease. I passed! Now, I just needed to convince my dad to let me borrow the car sometimes. Surprisingly, Dad was happy that I'd passed—I had been such a pain in his butt while learning to drive that he was relieved he no longer had to take me out every Saturday morning.

One of my closest friends in high school, Yvonne, died during this time. She had been born with some type of disorder that she'd never wanted to talk about, and I'd never asked since I did not want her to feel odd. After all, I knew what "odd" felt like. Yvonne was incredibly thin, and her face had several malformations. Her younger brother and mother looked "normal," so I was not sure if this was something genetic or sporadic, but to me, she was very beautiful. I loved her energy and how much she enjoyed life, but I had no clue about the demons she fought to stay alive. Even today, as a physician, I am not sure what her diagnosis was. Her funeral had a closed casket. I had not seen her for a few weeks before her death, so, at first, I was upset that it was closed. But the truth was that I wanted to remember her as someone full of life, not a body in a casket. I was a member of the glee club at that time, and at her funeral, we sang, "Soon and very soon, we are going to see the King." As I sang, I felt peace and happiness for Yvonne; she was going to see the King.

Nine

Loss of My Role Model

Yvonne was not the only person I lost in high school; my beloved Granny also died during this time. I knew she had diabetes. I knew she was on insulin. I knew she had problems with her sugars. That was as much as I understood back then. Now, as a physician, I know that there is a lot more to that story. If I had already been a doctor, I could have done something; I could have fixed her; I could have prevented her death. For a long time following her death, I had feelings of guilt. Granny did not have a poor diet and was admirably adherent to her diabetic regimen, but her diabetes was still uncontrollable. The failure to regulate sugars led to sugars in her urine, something that was routinely seen toward the end of her life.

Granny did a lot of the housework around the house, as both my mom and dad worked so that we could barely break even financially, and had been a tremendous help to us all. Without her helping at home, Mom and Dad could not make it through the workweek. The day before her death, Granny got up, made us breakfast, did chores, and had dinner waiting for us when we got home. She went to bed early that night, saying that she was exhausted. The next morning, my mom made us breakfast and said that she was going to have to call in sick so she could take Granny to the doctor. No one really explained anything to me; as far as I knew, she could have needed to go see the doctor because she had a common cold. So, our dad took us to school, which was typically dismissed midafternoon. That day, my dad showed up to school at midday and picked me up. When I inquired why he was picking me up so early, he did not give me any satisfactory explanation. I was mad with him because I was missing school to go on a joyride with him. For most kids, this would be awesome; for me, it was devastating. Additionally, he'd picked only *me* up, not my sisters or brother, so I was even more mad. I didn't understand why I was the only person to miss school while they got to stay until the end of the day! Dad finally confessed that he had picked them up earlier that morning but had left me in school since I had a big project that I'd wanted to present. He had returned to pick me up later to join my siblings, who were at the hospital with Granny. She was ill, and I needed to see her.

I got to the hospital and met my mom and siblings, who told me that Granny had passed away that morning. The only person who'd been with her was her daughter, my mom. My siblings had arrived much later, but I was the last person to know what was going on. My grandmother had gone to our family doctor that morning. She had a history of severe diabetes and presented with chest pain, shortness of breath, and extreme exhaustion. The doctor was suspicious of a heart attack and sent her via ambulance to the hospital, and, indeed, when she arrived, the studies confirmed that she was having a heart attack. Ultimately, what made her heart give out was a combination of the physical attributes of a heart attack and the emotional burden of knowing she was having one. My mom said she expired shortly after arriving at the hospital and learning what was happening. Things happened so fast that not even Mom had the opportunity to say goodbye. I walked over to her lifeless body; she looked so peaceful. I wanted to reach out to hug her, but I was afraid to feel her cold, motionless body. I held it together very well, refusing to cry. It was Granny who had taught me how to be a strong woman, and I did not want to disappoint her. Even though I just stood there for what felt like hours, it was maybe only minutes that I stood, staring, not knowing how much more to say than, "I love you and will miss you."

After Granny's death, my parents spoke to the hospital officials, and then we headed home. The ride home was silent, as none of us wanted to say anything. We were all in shock, wondering how our lives would continue without her. She'd been such an integral part of our day-to-day lives. Granny had taught me self-assurance. I'd learned from her that even though I was a tiny Asian girl, I could still do anything in life that I wanted—but I had to be willing to work for it. As a child, I used to snuggle with her at nights when I could not fall asleep. Who would I go to now with all my fears? She'd had the answer to all my problems. I was still so naïve and needed her wisdom to educate me about real life.

Our church was and still is a small community, in which we had a close relationship with everyone. Pastor Johnson personally came by our home that night to pray with us, and it was during his prayer that I finally let go and started crying. I felt the salted tears roll down my cheeks, my eyes red and inflamed, my nasal passage completely congested because I could not get everything out fast enough. As we held hands during Pastor Johnson's prayer, my hands trembled in his because I could not control the unbearable loss that I was experiencing. The more he prayed, the more I cried. His words echoed in every beat of my heart. Pastor Johnson stayed for a long time, consoling us and then making arrangements with my parents. Granny had passed away on a Thursday, and they planned for a Tuesday funeral.

We kids went to school on Friday. Everyone knew what had happened; it is amazing how quickly news gets around in small communities. Almost everyone I encountered that day came up to me to offer condolences. My parents were busy figuring out which casket to buy, what dress Granny should wear, etc. . . . Then Tuesday rolled around. We had gone to the church earlier that morning to make sure everything was ready before the funeral started. Pastor Johnson, always such a good public speaker, delivered an amazing speech. His words resonated with me that day because I knew that Granny was going to a better place. The funeral home had done a fantastic job with the presentation—she looked so beautiful, wearing a rose-colored dress as she lay in her casket. Like an angel. She was the most beautiful woman I had ever known, and she had not lost any of her beauty, even in death. At the burial ground, I watched as the casket was lowered six feet deep and then the first shovel of dirt was placed on it. I knew at that moment that was the last time I would see my Granny.

The deaths of Yvonne, Granny, and my sisters Nikki and Andromeda are some of the factors that influenced me to become a physician. It occurred to me numerous times that if I had been a doctor, I could have saved them. To this day, I still remember the chill I felt going down my spine as I saw Nikki's tiny casket go six feet under. Losing Andromeda on my eighth birthday and watching my mom struggle with the subsequent pregnancy certainly made me more partial to taking care of women and children. But Granny's death hit me the hardest. I was fifteen when she passed away, and I had grown to know and love her all those fifteen years. She was my role model. She'd had the answer to everything. She would have wanted me to pursue my education and make something of myself.

Ten

The College Years

I applied to several colleges toward the end of high school. To tell the truth, while I was inclined to do medicine, I did not have enough exposure to make a definitive decision regarding exactly what I wanted to do with my life. I beat myself up for not having a plan, but I was only sixteen when I graduated from high school, and there are not many sixteen-year-olds who know exactly what they want to do with their lives. However, I knew that I was good at math and sciences, so I applied under the engineering program at some colleges and the biology program at others. Eventually, I went to college at the University of the Virgin Islands (UVI) in St. Thomas under their biology program.

My parents felt that I was too young to be so far away—the mainland was certainly too far—and that the other programs were still too expensive despite some scholarships. Sure enough, they packed up and moved from St. Croix to St. Thomas so I did not have to live on my own. My younger sister Marie was just a year behind me, in the eleventh grade. St. Dunstan's Episcopal School had closed after I graduated since the church could no longer afford to keep the school open. Many of the eleventh graders had problems transferring to other schools, so some of them, including my sister, took twelfth grade over the summer break, allowing them to graduate early. My sister attended UVI part time in the fall and then matriculated full time in the spring, so we were now in many classes together. She, too, did not know what she wanted to do with her life, so she decided to major in biology too.

In our second month on St. Thomas, my mom started having such massive hemorrhaging that her skin became pale. It takes a lot of blood loss to make a brown person look white. After she passed out in the kitchen from dizziness, we rushed her to the hospital. Due to her six pregnancies, Mom had always seen a doctor. Her youngest child, my brother, was just about to celebrate his fifth birthday, but she still saw a gynecologist yearly and knew she had fibroids. However, I do not think my mother understood exactly what fibroids were or that, in some cases, they can cause severe bleeding and pain. Her blood count was low when she presented to the emergency room that day. She needed a transfusion. My father and mother are the same blood type, so Dad insisted that the staff take a pint of blood from him to give to my mother, which they did. My parents are typical Asian parents: there is no public display of affection. But, every so often, I see in them a love that will transcend time. The truth is that they have been together so long that the thought of living without the other would be hard, even if they do not want to admit to this publicly. Now, when they argue, my mom always says that she is senseless because her husband's blood runs through her veins. They are the funniest cranky old couple and still very much in love. Once my mom was transfused and discharged, she made an appointment with the doctor who had done her cesarean section. As she was so attached to this doctor and trusted him with her life, she flew back to Antigua to have him do her hysterectomy. Once again, Mom received outstanding care.

During my first year of college, I found other activities to keep me busy. I worked at the Kinney's shoe store on St. Thomas to make a few extra dollars; additionally, I volunteered at the local hospital. I was just a college freshman; therefore, my duties were very simple at the hospital. I first underwent an introductory course, which involved learning how to properly wash your hands. They did not have the alcohol-based hand sanitizers that we currently have now, so I learned how to wash my hands the old-school way: I had to turn on the faucet, dampen my hands, apply soap, rub in the soap thoroughly on the entire surface area of my hands for at least twenty seconds, rinse, wipe with a towel, and then use the towel to turn the faucet off. We had to do this before and after interacting with each patient. *Whenever in doubt, wash your hands again.* My duties in the hospital wards consisted mainly of helping patients ambulate, making sure their water jugs were filled, and sitting with the elderly.

When I arrived at the hospital, I'd go to the volunteer desk, where I'd receive a ward assignment. This was my first introduction to a hospital, and I felt needed by the patients and useful to others.

My parents stayed less than one year in St. Thomas before moving back to St. Croix because they missed their home and friends there. My sister and I then lived together in an apartment on St. Thomas; the landlords lived on the second floor, we lived in one apartment on the first floor, and a young couple lived in the other apartment. When our parents left us, I was eighteen, taking care of my seventeen-year-old sister. While we were living alone, another major hurricane came along. Hurricane Marilyn left St. Thomas with the same devastation as Hurricane Hugo had St. Croix just years prior. My sister and I made it through by hiding in the closet, which was the safest place in the apartment, for everything had happened so quickly that we had not had any time to get a flight to St. Croix. The winds were too strong, and the airport had already shut down commercial flights long before the hurricane hit. We thought that since we had done this before, we would be OK, but there was just one problem: we were kids with no resources.

As Hurricane Marilyn passed, we heard loud wind and heavy rain; then we heard the shatter of glass upstairs. The second floor, which had beautiful floor-to-ceiling glass windows, was being severely damaged. We heard our landlords scurrying to various parts of the house while we shook with fear in the closet, thinking we were about to die. My sister and I had a close relationship, but, in the closet, we apologized for any wrongdoing we had caused the other. The next day, after the hurricane had passed, we came out to see what had happened. The entire second floor had been demolished, so that the house appeared to be only one story after the hurricane. Although the other apartment on the first floor had severe damage and broken windows, our apartment did not have any damage! We surely had guardian angels looking over us that day!

Our building was in the hills, with very few neighbors, so we felt like we were stranded on a deserted island with no resources or people. At least we had each other. The entire island had been wiped out as far as we could see. However, we did like we always did: we figured out a way to survive. Luckily, we had a gas stove, so we started cooking the food in the fridge, figuring that we would work on the cans in the pantry later. We had enough bottled water to last for only a few days, and we were worried what would happen to us after that. Fortunately, we found a pipe in the yard and used this to bring water in by bucket so we could flush the toilet and bathe. On the third day following the hurricane, I heard a man's footsteps outside our apartment. No one knew we were there, so, at first, I was afraid, but as the footsteps drew closer, I recognized the footstep pattern. It was our father! Fear suddenly became relief, for now there was someone older and more responsible to take care of things. By then, there were small charter planes, able to hold eight people at most, flying between St. Croix and St. Thomas. My dad had found a way to buy a plane ticket to St. Thomas and three tickets back to St. Croix. I am sure it cost him a small fortune, and I still do not know how he found us that quickly. The roads were terrible from all the debris and damaged homes. Nothing was recognizable. It would have been very easy to overlook our building or know that there were survivors there. When we arrived at our home in St. Croix, I let out a huge sigh of relief. St. Croix had also been severely damaged and was without power, but my parents had stocked up on supplies and already had the generator running. We were now in a location a lot more habitable than St. Thomas.

Not all of college was terrible; there were lots of fun courses. We were required to take four physical education classes to graduate, so I signed up for a tae kwon do elective. Just like dance, I fell in love with tae kwon do. The teacher noticed how much I enjoyed the class and invited me to join his tae kwon do school outside of the university course. I never made it to black belt, but at just over one hundred pounds, I was a pretty darn good blue belt. Another elective that I decided to take was swimming. I will be the first to admit that despite growing up on an island, I'd never learned how to swim until then. A lot of it had to do with my parents not knowing how to swim, meaning they could never teach us. They made us very fearful of the water because, if we went out too deep at the beach, they were afraid that they would not be able to swim out to save us. The swimming class in college took place at the beach in the ocean water. No, there was no swimming pool when we had a body of water surrounding an island. There were two other women in the class who were also learning to swim, so the instructor had us spend the first half of the semester swimming in the shallow waters and perfecting all the strokes. Our midterm was to make sure we could do all the swim strokes, which I accomplished quite well. The second half of the semester was spent swimming out in the deep water. I was excellent at the strokes, but one good thing about being in shallow water is that when I was tired, I could just stand up. The first time I went out in the deep, I learned that out there, on the contrary, I could *not* do that. You see, I got tired swimming and reflexively thought I could stand, but the water was too deep. Yes, I was drowning. Luckily, one of my classmates, who was like a fish and was just taking the class for fun, was nearby. He pulled me up. The instructor, a hard-core ex-military man, was mad at me. Instead of trying to gently help me overcome my fears, he decided that for the rest of the semester, I would spend the entire one-hour class doing laps out in the deep waters. I did fine, but it was amazing how, once I mentally overcame the fear, the physical activity became so easy.

We had been living in the US Virgin Islands for many years; we had our green cards and were now eligible for citizenship via naturalization. My parents completed the applications. Apart from myself, all my parents' children were under the age of eighteen, so once my parents naturalized, my siblings automatically naturalized too. However, I had to take the civics test, interview, and ultimately the naturalization ceremony on my own. It was not difficult. I had to memorize several questions and answers about the United States' government and history, which only took a few minutes to review since I knew the answers to most of them from high school courses. I learned during that time that there were many American citizens, born on American soil, who did not know very basic US government and history. I did the fingerprints, took my two-by-two picture, and went in for the ceremony, feeling proud to now be a US citizen.

Eleven

Transitioning from College to Medical School

I enjoyed my first couple of years in college, yet I still kept thoughts of pursuing medicine in the back of my mind. In the fall of my sophomore year, two doctors from Boston University School of Medicine (BUSM) came down to UVI to visit. BUSM had both seven-year and eight-year programs (college and medical school combined) for students matriculated at the undergraduate campus of Boston University. They were now looking to add several other colleges to a similar eight-year program that they called the Early Medical School Selection Program (EMSSP), and since Boston was already cold by November, they enjoyed coming down to the Virgin Islands at this time of year to recruit new students. I had done research with a marine biologist at UVI who knew I had fantastic grades and wanted to go places in life, and he highly recommended that I speak with these two doctors. One of the men from BUSM was now turning over the program to the other, so I met both men just before my eighteenth birthday. It was not an interview—just an introduction—but I decided to apply to the program. My application was flawless except for one major error: I typed a well-crafted cover letter but misspelled one of their names. It was a typographical error, as I knew his name very well. I was about to fax it when I had it reviewed by a professor at UVI, who quickly caught the mistake and made me change it. Thank goodness! Incorrectly spelling the name of the program director would not have left a good impression. One of the marine biology professors reviewed my personal essay. Since writing such an essay was natural for me, the words came out so easily. I wrote about my sister Andromeda, her death on my birthday, and my desire to become a doctor so that I could help women have healthy babies. When my sister Marie heard that I was applying to the EMSSP program, she also applied, and we were both granted interviews.

In the spring of my sophomore year, we flew to Boston for the interview. Everyone was so nice and sophisticated. Despite the fact that I was a kid from an island and felt a bit out of place (even though, on paper, I was highly qualified), I did fine on the interview by just being myself. Following the interviews, I had massive nausea and vomiting, and everyone kept asking me if I was OK. Many thought that I had bombed the interview, but I had actually caught a terrible gastrointestinal bug. Still, I felt the interviews went well. However, if other people thought that my symptoms were related to the interview, I questioned whether the interviewers might have thought this too. Although the symptoms did not start until late afternoon, well after the interviews, we had a final dinner that evening, at which others heard that I had been sick that afternoon. Now, I was worried. It was unnecessary worry, though: both my sister and I were accepted into the EMSSP program.

Even though I did not know it back then, my acceptance into that program opened a world of opportunities for me that otherwise I would not have had. There are not enough words in my vocabulary to describe how grateful I am to the amazing UVI professors who provided extraordinary guidance to an impressionable kid like myself, as well as to the many other incredible people in my life who took the time to invest in me. I owe so much to them. However, acceptance into the EMSSP program was only a conditional acceptance for medical school. As part of the program, I would spend the summer between my sophomore and junior years, the summer between my junior and senior years, and my entire senior year at Boston University, taking some college courses but also some modular courses that would count toward my medical school curriculum. Depending on how well I did in these courses, I would be granted full admission to BUSM after my senior year. In addition, I was still required to also take the Medical College Admission Test (MCAT) before starting BUSM. The credits from the courses that I took through the program were transferred back to UVI so I could graduate from that university at the end of my senior year.

The courses at Boston University were different than they were at UVI. For example, I was now in larger classes; many times, I could only see the professor and "chalkboard" from a projector screen, which was very different from the smaller classes at UVI, where all the professors knew my name and face. At UVI, I knew all my classmates very well; some of them were like brothers and sisters to me. But at Boston University, I was just another student in a large classroom. In many ways, I felt like a small-town girl who had now moved to the big city. In Boston, I had to learn how to use the subway—"the T"—and take elevators to high floors in tall skyscrapers. At UVI, my sister and I lived in an apartment; in Boston, we lived in a school dormitory on Commonwealth Avenue and Bay State Road, with the bathrooms located down the hall from our room. It was my first time learning how to wear a robe and walk down the hall to use a common bathroom. During my senior year, however, I got lucky and stayed in a dormitory building for graduate students. Everyone was very nice. One of my roommates took me under her wing like a big sister to show me the ropes. She was the oldest of three girls, so it was natural for her to guide me. My course load was very heavy, but, occasionally, I would go with her to her church and spend time with her friends. I had my twentieth birthday in Boston, and my roommate made my birthday super special: she invited all her friends in the building to throw me a surprise party. It was truly a surprise. Her friendship alone was more than I could have asked for.

Unfortunately, my first winter in Boston, I came down with the flu. I had never received the flu shot in St. Croix since contracting it during winters there was rare. This was my first experience with the flu. My kind roomie, another angel that God had sent my way, helped me get over it. I went to her wedding several years later, and we are still friends today.

My first full year in Boston was exciting but also intimidating. We ate at the school cafeteria instead of cooking in our apartment, as we did at UVI; it was so much fun trying out different cuisines in the cafeteria. That winter, the winter of 1996, I had my first experience with snow and bitter cold, I bought my first official winter outfit: coat, hat, gloves, boots, thick socks, scarf, and earmuffs. One of the other students told me about Filene's Basement, where my sister and I were able to purchase items inexpensively. Winter was a lot of fun for a while, but I surely wished for summer to come around soon. I had spent all my life on an island wanting to get off it because there was not enough opportunity, but after my first winter in Boston, I understood why the US Virgin Islands and many other tropical islands are often referred to as paradise. When I was at UVI, I swam for exercise, but it was too cold to swim in Boston, so I started running. This was my first experience with running, an activity that is now an addiction. Boston University undergraduate campus is on one side of the Charles River, and on the other side is Cambridge. The Massachusetts Institute of Technology (MIT) and Harvard campuses are in Cambridge, so I would run along the Charles River, cross Massachusetts Avenue, take the Harvard Bridge into Cambridge, and wander my way back. It was fantastic exercise and an opportunity to discover my new environment.

In the spring of our senior year, it became very real that my sister and I would matriculate into BUSM the following fall, as we had been lucky enough to now be fully accepted to medical school. There was just one problem: How were we going to pay for this? Tuition was very high, and we also needed money for room and board, books, and other small necessities. I started looking at the options. Several students had told us about military scholarships, through which later, as physicians, we would repay the scholarships by serving time at various military facilities and assignments. We applied for the navy's Health Professions Scholarship Program (HPSP), but my sister got accepted before I did. I was too underweight to be in the military, so I needed to bulk up. It was so much fun going to the cafeteria and eating lots of ice cream (one of my many favorite desserts) to gain a few pounds in order to be accepted into the program. My sister and I returned briefly to St. Thomas for graduation in May 1997, at which I graduated summa cum laude with a bachelor of science in biology. Although it was a lot of work, I felt such a sense of accomplishment. I was now ready for the next step on my career path.

Twelve

Medical School

In the late summer of 1997, we started medical school at BUSM, moving from Boston University's undergraduate campus to be closer to the medical school. We rented a small apartment on Harrison Avenue, close to the medical center, so we could walk to classes. BUSM does a white-coat ceremony for each matriculating class at the beginning of the school year; we were so excited to wear a white coat and take the Hippocratic oath.

One of our classes that first semester was anatomy. My mom, being from a very traditional upbringing, was scared for us to be in a room with dead bodies. We were already scientists, however, and were extraordinarily grateful for the human beings who had donated their bodies so we could learn. There were approximately 150 students in the class, with groups of 6 students assigned to each cadaver. My sister and I were in separate groups, which worked out well since it allowed us to teach each other from our different dissections. The human body is amazing; we are all the same species but so different in personality and in the characterization of our bodies. We are truly individuals in many ways.

The dissections took a long time, even with six students in each group; many times, we returned to the lab after dinner to finish our work. When you thought you had everything memorized on your cadaver, you would go to another group's dissection and try to find the same structures, which was a great way to get to know our classmates. That was one of many examples of BUSM students' sportsmanship, a motto highly encouraged by the university, which also encouraged group activities and teamwork. I also joined a study group, which was critical, as there was no way you could get through all the necessary material without support. We went to classes from 8:00 a.m. to 5:00 p.m. every day, and then we kept each other awake at night, studying. Our breaks were stopping for lunch and dinner or running to the corner store for Mountain Dew. There was a time I wished I could just hook myself up to intravenous Mountain Dew! Above all, we had to stay up long hours to get our studying completed.

The summer following my first year at medical school, I attended the navy's Officer Indoctrination School (OIS) in Newport, Rhode Island. One of my classmates was kind enough to give me a ride to this very intense six weeks of learning how to be a naval officer. We learned how to make our beds, have tidy uniforms, salute, and march, along with pretty much everything else that the military needed us to know. Of necessity, we woke up at ridiculous early hours to do physical training (PT) before breakfast, with more PT in the afternoons and evenings. I learned terminology like "the head" for the bathroom and "mess hall" for the cafeteria. During training, they taught us lifesaving water skills, but you had to already know how to swim and tread water before applying these skills. Thank goodness I had learned to swim a few years earlier! I clearly remember one activity in which we had to jump off a fairly high diving board into the deep water of the swimming pool. I was very nervous the first time I did this, but I closed my eyes and took a big leap of faith off the board. I splashed into the water and then had to swim back up to the surface. I did fine even though I felt that my heart was going to jump out of my chest from all the anticipation. We interacted with more senior officers to learn what life was like in the military and how they'd made military careers for themselves. OIS was designed for all officers in training regardless of what core or field they were pursuing, so we had a diverse blend of career interests.

I returned from OIS with still four more weeks to go before our second year would start. One of my BUSM classmates and I had already made arrangements to travel to Guatemala on our own— we were going to live with a family in Antigua and study Spanish, and we planned to volunteer at hospitals in Guatemala City and in Antigua. We booked our trip through a Spanish learning school in Antigua and figured that once we arrived, we would be able to investigate volunteer opportunities at hospitals and clinics. Since we had only one year of medical school under our belts, our lack of experience would not allow us to do too much clinical work. Still, this was a great way for us to get to know each other, as we were in the same class of 150 students. We had spoken often but did not know each other well. Our plane ride to Guatemala City was uneventful, and the school had ordered a van to pick us up at the airport. We each stayed with a different family, not realizing that we would not be together until that night, when the van dropped us off at the families' front doors. Despite the separation, we felt safe, and everyone was nice and welcoming. My companion's host family lived just a five-minute walk from my host family, so whenever we felt lonely and wanted a break to talk in English, we walked over to the other's dwelling. The families' homes were intriguing, as I had not seen these types of homes before. Each had a central courtyard with the house built around it. We had all three meals with the family, and I so enjoyed the Guatemalan cooking. I spoke Spanish to the family during the meals; they were always interested in what I'd done that day. Of course, explaining it to them in Spanish was a challenge. Mornings Monday through Friday were tied up with one-on-one tutoring with a Spanish teacher, and in the afternoons, we walked around Antigua as tourists. One of our favorite spots was the central park area just outside of the Santa Catalina Arch, which was busy with vendors and people strolling through. It was our favorite spot to watch people and really take in the culture. I bought so much colorful clothing and beaded jewelry from the local vendors, all of it made by hand. My friend and I volunteered several times at the local hospital in Antigua, delivering very basic services like helping patients ambulate. We took a trip to Guatemala City one afternoon and volunteered similarly in the hospital wards there, but the trip was a bit expensive and not as safe as the van used by the Spanish-speaking school, so we never returned to Guatemala City.

During the afternoons, the two of us planned our weekends since we did not have Spanish classes during the weekends and the weekends were perfect for long trips. My companion was excellent at the touristy stuff: she did research and planned a lot of our weekends, and during the week, she asked the locals for the best and safest places to buy tickets to and visit. She wanted us to see the highlights of Guatemala and the neighboring countries before leaving. I am grateful for her planning because, otherwise, I would have been content with sitting around Antigua every weekend.

Our first weekend trip was to see the Mayan ruins in Tikal, which were magnificent. We couldn't imagine how the Mayans had built these giant structures so long ago without all the modern-day construction equipment that we have today! The Mayans were truly advanced in their intellectual, mathematical, astronomical, and artistic skills. We climbed every ruin that the tour guide allowed us to, which was not only fascinating but great exercise. I was grateful that I had just completed the grueling physical training of OIS—it was the only way I could keep up with my athletic friend, who was in excellent physical condition and full of so much energy. The following weekend, we went to Copán in Honduras, where, similarly, we visited the Mayan ruins. Once again, they were magical.

Our last free weekend, we planned to climb Volcán Pacaya, but my friend was not feeling well toward the end of that week, so I had to go on the trip by myself. Because there were other tourists going along, I did not feel unsafe. Volcán Pacaya is an active complex volcano that rises 8,373 feet above sea level. I got off the tour bus and, along with my fellow tourists, followed our group's local tour guide assigned to take us up the volcano. I was twenty-one years old at that time, and the guide looked like he was in his early sixties. He was a thin, athletic man who carried a long stick like a staff and was in better athletic condition than I was despite being decades older than me. He climbed Volcán Pacaya five days a week and made it look easy. The first part of the climb up was manageable, like climbing any other mountain, but the second part of the climb involved climbing up ashes. For every two steps up, we slipped back one. When we finally got to the top, I saw the red molten rocks and lava flow. It was steamy and hot up there—so steamy that my cheap student camera kept fogging up. None of the pictures I took that day did justice to what I saw with my eyes, but it was astounding. For a brief moment, I felt fear: this volcano had small spurts of activity, and I wondered whether I was putting my life in danger. Despite the fear, I was really happy that I'd made it up to the top, as some of the older tourists had abbreviated their climb earlier on. Going down was more challenging than climbing up because we were literally sliding down the ashes. For every step downward, my foot skidded two more steps. Our weekend excursions were life changing. We flew back to Boston the next weekend, our Spanish vocabulary and sentence structure much improved. We now had a larger appreciation for another culture and the wonders of the world.

While I was in Newport, Rhode Island, and Antigua, Guatemala, I sublet my room to another student. She really liked my sister and I and became our roommate in our second year. We had to move to a bigger apartment in the same building, but it made the rent easier when split three ways. Our friend was an amazingly likeable person—everyone who met her loved her. She, her mom—who has a bigger-than-life personality—and I loved to dance. Once in a while, we went to a club and just danced until the club closed, but we never drank alcohol since dancing was already a drug for us. Our former roommate and I are still in contact today; every time I am in Boston, I always have dinner with her and her family. Her four children are just as perfect as she is.

My second year of medical school was uneventful. We had very long hours, with more attending classes during the days and studying at nights; medical school was all I knew. In the mornings, I started running with one of my girlfriends, which was a way that I could relieve stress. We ran in the hot summers and the frigid winters. Although we only ran for about thirty minutes, it was enough to get the heart pumping and the mind clear. On Friday nights, I attended tae kwon do, my small gift to myself as something I enjoyed doing. I did not have classes for medical school on Saturdays, so I allowed myself one night off. Giving myself these stress-relieving breaks made my focus on studying sharper. We studied at all opportunities; sometimes, we went to other school campuses while studying just to have a change of scenery and break up the monotony. If we knew students from other schools, they would help us get into their school's library so we could study there. It was like taking a field trip without feeling guilty that we were not studying.

During my second year of medical school, I started volunteering at soup kitchens, senior homes, and drives that donated winter clothing and basic medical care to the very unfortunate. While I was not yet a full-fledged doctor, I felt that I was helping people. In truth, I got more out of the volunteer experience than the person I was helping. I also volunteered at a women's clinic that provided basic care to women in need and attended several seminars at domestic shelters to learn how to identify these women, who often do not have a voice for themselves. Additionally, I volunteered at the call center for a women's shelter; seeing women and children suffer was a difficult and heart-wrenching experience. Nauseated as I listened to their difficult stories, I asked myself why the world wasn't kinder to helpless women and children. This experience further influenced my decision to become an advocate for women and children by pursuing obstetrics, gynecology, and ultimately fertility. I continued to learn a lot about humanity from these experiences. It is amazing that what I'd learned in church and in school sometimes did not apply to real life; it became clear that people wanted me to meet them where they were.

At the end of our second year, we were required to take the US Medical Licensing Examination (USMLE). The USMLE was a standardized test that all medical students in the country took. It was important because residency programs looked at this standardized score when deciding which students to accept. The exam was divided into three steps: one taken at the end of the second year, one taken some time in the fourth year, and the third taken some time in residency. Typically, students took the test at a computerized test-taking center. Obtaining a good score was important, so, needless to say, everyone was stressed—more stressed even than during the last two years of studying. I did well, which was a big burden removed from my shoulders as we finished the second year of medical school and rolled straight into the third year. There was no summer vacation for us; the previous year had been our last summer vacation for the rest of our lives.

At that time, the third and fourth years of medical school at BUSM were all clinical rotations. The third year included the core fields of medicine that all students had to rotate through, and the fourth year was mostly elective clinical rotations. I started my third year with obstetrics and gynecology. Generally, you should not start your third year with the field of medicine that you will eventually choose. Typically, you should rotate through that field toward the end of the year, when your clinical skills and knowledge are more adept, but I was way too excited to start in obstetrics and gynecology. I wanted to know whether it was the right field for me. One day in the obstetrics ward, they called for a doctor to deliver a baby; the patient was actively pushing. The nurse was in the room with the patient. All the "real" doctors were already tied up in other deliveries and surgeries. It was just us students hanging out at the nursing station when I heard the call for a doctor and ran to the room. I quickly put on a sterile gown and got ready for the delivery, thinking that a "real" doctor would follow me in shortly. The patient delivered so quickly that I was the only person there, but everything went smoothly. Thank goodness, the patient had had babies before, which made the delivery very easy. It was only after I was done with the delivery that I realized I was in the room without a doctor supervising—another experience that influenced my decision to take care of women and children. It gave me great gratification to know that I made a difference in someone's life. My next rotations were internal medicine, surgery, pediatrics, psychology, and family medicine. I can say that I truly enjoyed all specialties of medicine, but, in the end, I chose obstetrics/gynecology for many reasons: it was the field that had initially attracted me to medicine, it would allow me to take care of women, and it was a nice blend of medicine and surgery.

I had an even bigger appreciation for human life after my third year of medical school. One of the emotionally difficult rotations for me was my internal medicine rotation at the Veterans Administration (VA) hospital, where there were men and women who had put their lives on the line in the past—true heroes, in my eyes. They were now ill and needed help. Some were critically ill. Those were the ones that I remember so well. Two particular patients come to mind, one a veteran who had a severe case of adult leukemia. He was in an isolated room since he was prone to infections and would get sick if exposed to others, and he was taking many toxic medications but not getting well. I knew very little about him, but I noticed he never had visitors even though there were family members' names and numbers in his chart. Surely I was the most consistent person in his life. This man saw me at least four times per day for my scheduled rounds, and sometimes I would stop by just to see if he wanted to chat with someone. He had end-stage disease, and it was only a matter of time. I had to draw blood on my patient daily to measure his blood count. His veins were not good due to a combination of the toxic chemotherapy that he had received and the many blood draws and intravenous lines that he had had. Because the only good veins left were in his feet, I drew blood from his feet regularly. He had been my patient for about two weeks when I came in to work one morning and found his room now occupied by someone else. He had passed away the night before. Although I had lost many family members in my life, every death sends emotional pain through my body. I had known he was in the end stage, but I had not been ready for this. The resident physician who worked with me on this patient saw how much I was grieving and sat down to talk with me. This was the first patient that I had lost. That physician gave me a reality pep talk: I needed to learn how to separate work from emotion. The other patient that I recall was a cranky old guy who had smoked tobacco and drunk alcohol for a great portion of his life. Despite his crankiness, he was still very human, hiding a lot of pain under his cranky behavior. He presented with bloody vomiting and fevers of unknown origin. A full evaluation revealed that he had throat cancer, so he was then transferred from our service to the cancer service. When I left the VA, I heard that he was doing well.

Thirteen

The Event That Changed My Entire Life

Toward the end of my third year of medical school, I sent a formal request asking the school to allow me to do my fourth year over two years, as I was interested in setting up some international rotations. Several students in previous years had done so, and they shared with me the physician contacts who had helped them travel to underserved areas in other countries. This would be a perfect way for me to get some hands-on experience while serving areas of the world that otherwise would not have help. Since I was now more clinically proficient than when I'd visited Guatemala after my first year of medical school, I was particularly interested in going to Mexico and to Central and South America. I have always enjoyed working with the Hispanic population; it would also be a great way for me to practice my Spanish. After my sister realized that I was going to take a year off, she did the same.

We could not afford to stay in the apartment on Harrison Avenue since we would have to pay an extra year of rent, so we moved to Jamaica Plain. There, we found a three-family house in which the owner lived on the third floor. There were already tenants on the first floor, so we moved in on the second floor. Our roommate did not move with us because she planned to graduate at the end of our fourth year, so we found another roommate to take the third room in the apartment. Our new apartment, however, was not within walking distance of the school. Hence, we decided to buy a used car. Instead of going to a car dealership and negotiating, we started to look at ads. We called the phone number in an ad for a used Toyota Camry and luckily connected with a sweet man who was selling his wife's car because he wanted to surprise her with a newer model. The Camry was still in excellent condition, and the transaction was uneventful. Now I had to learn how to maintain a car and drive in the wintery weather.

My first winter with the vehicle, I had to shovel the car out of two feet of snow several times, so I began regularly buying large bags of rock salt from the store to help melt the ice and snow. I also bought a defroster that I could put in the keyhole if it ever froze up and prevented me from entering. One day, I left the hospital to go home and realized that I was incredibly low on gas. I stopped at the gas station on the way home and got out of the car to pump. There was one problem: the cover to the gas tank was frozen over and would not open, despite me releasing the lever from inside the car. I had to use the ice scraper to break up the ice in the crevices between the car and the gas cover before I could finally unscrew the gas cap. There were new experiences to learn from quite frequently.

As part of my HPSP program, I needed to do a few rotations in the navy. I chose to do a sports medicine rotation at their location in Annapolis, Maryland, where the Naval Academy is located. I was going to work at the sports medicine clinic. It was a beautiful August; since Annapolis is near the water, I had planned to take lots of walks along the piers and eat good seafood in my free time. Knowing that I wanted to do obstetrics/gynecology (OB-GYN), I decided that most of my elective rotations would be in other fields. I wanted to learn more about general medicine before I specialized; additionally, a sports medicine rotation could be quite useful since I was in the military and also very physically active myself.

One Thursday afternoon at the clinic, we were told that the next morning, we would go to the hospital to observe a surgery. The plan was to meet at the clinic and all take a small van to the hospital. As we boarded the van Friday morning, there were several attending physicians, residents, and students present. Attending physicians are doctors who have completed their training in a specialized field. Residents are physicians who are in training in a specific medical field. Students are still in medical school, working toward their graduate degree. We estimated that we would arrive at the hospital early, so we stopped at Starbucks. I ordered a tall black iced coffee, most of which was ice with very little coffee. As we were approaching the hospital, we received a call that the surgery had been canceled; therefore, we turned around and headed back to the clinic. There was lots of small talk in the van during this time. When we arrived at the clinic in Annapolis, I was sitting in the back and was one of the last people to exit. I got off the van but could not walk, was weak, and had no control over my muscles or balance. I do not recall what happened next.

I woke up in one of the clinic beds, disoriented and unable to recall what had happened. How had I gotten there? I thought it was Saturday but was told that it was still Friday. I spied a plastic mug of water and cup at my bedside, and since I was thirsty, the physician's assistant (PA) who was with me told me that I could have some water. When I looked over again, now there were two cups and two mugs—I had double vision. I glanced back at the PA. Two of him were sitting right next to each other. This was not good. I also had blurry vision, so I asked for my glasses, hoping that everything would seem normal once I was wearing them. The glasses did not correct the double or blurry vision. I told the PA but insisted on pouring my own water. I was an independent woman; I could pour my own glass of water. So, I poured, but I missed the glass. Looking over at the PA, I knew something was wrong. Because I am left handed, I held the mug in my left hand. When I attempted to hold the cup with my right hand, I had no motor control over it, as if my hand had fallen asleep, and my right arm felt like deadweight, like the feeling you get when you lie on one arm too long at night. I asked if I could get up to go to the restroom, but when I attempted to get up, I could neither feel nor move my right leg. I asked the PA whether there was something wrong with my face; the left half felt like it was falling. Now I was really scared. I had never lost control over my body. At twenty-three years of age, I was in the best shape of my life. I had well-defined musculature, including a six-pack, and I was an amazing runner and dancer. Additionally, I had never drunk alcohol, smoked tobacco, or tried any form of drugs. If you take good care of your health, you should never get sick. At least, that is what I thought!

Confused, I asked the physician assistant what had happened. He said that I had passed out when I got off the van and that one of the residents had caught me before I could hit the concrete ground. They had brought me in for monitoring; my vital signs were good despite being unresponsive. I was breathing but appeared to be in a deep sleep, unable to be roused. The doctors checked my sugar level and found that it was not abnormally elevated or depressed. Like every morning, I had eaten breakfast that day, and I therefore had a normal blood sugar level. What, then, was the source of my symptoms—double and blurry vision, left-side facial drooping, and complete right hemiparesis (no ability to move any part of the right side of my body from the neck down)? I attempted to go to the bathroom again, determined that whatever this was, I was going to beat it. So, I stood up and wobbled to the bathroom, walking like a drunk as I dragged one side of my body. Because I was in such good physical shape and had a very determined personality, I masked my symptoms by forcing myself to pull through this, convinced that I would be able to do so.

The clinic was a small outpatient sports medicine clinic, so the doctors sent me to a nearby imaging center for a computed tomography (CT) scan of my head. The scan was negative for any bleeds in the brain. By this time, it was late Friday evening, and everyone in the clinic was getting ready to go home. I was just finishing my first week of this rotation and did not know anyone in Annapolis; however, one of the senior doctors did not want me to stay by myself, so he took me to his house, where I stayed with him and his family that evening. I did not know what was going on back then, but despite my normal CT scan, he still felt something was very wrong with me. The next day, he took me to another imaging center for a magnetic resonance imaging (MRI) of my brain. Since it was Saturday, we had to wait until Monday for a radiologist to read my MRI. Feeling guilty being a burden to him and his family, I told him that I should be OK staying in my hotel room that night. If there was a problem, I had his cell phone number and would call him. My vision and facial dropping had improved, but I still walked like a drunk. I got back to my hotel room and called my parents in St. Croix, explaining everything and assuring them that I was OK and that this was sure to pass. The day before (Friday) had been my parents' anniversary, and that day (Saturday) was my mom's birthday. I apologized for not calling on Friday—I hadn't wanted to worry them.

Monday morning, I took a cab to the sports medicine clinic, where my rental car was still parked. When I arrived, the physician who'd taken me in on Friday came to me and informed me that my MRI was abnormal and they were going to send me to Walter Reed National Military Medical Center to be admitted for a full evaluation. After my arrival at Walter Reed, I was checked in to the neurology service. This was the first time that I had ever been a patient in a hospital before, so it was all new to me. The good news is that, three days after they began, all my symptoms were gone, and I fortunately did not feel helpless like I had on Friday. When the senior neurology resident came in to speak with me, he explained that my MRI showed an abnormality and informed me that either I had had a stroke on Friday or this was my first attack of multiple sclerosis (MS). When I heard MS, I felt my heart sink—I knew that MS was a debilitating disease. Not that a stroke was any better news than MS, though!

After multiple imaging studies and laboratory testing, it was determined that I had had a stroke. The lesion was not too far from my breathing center (the area of the brain responsible for breathing). A stroke at the breathing center of my brain would have caused acute death. Now that I had a diagnosis, the biggest question was how a healthy twenty-three-year-old could have had a stroke. More imaging studies and laboratory tests were scheduled. The staff drained multiple tubes of blood from me daily, and I was tested for all forms of infectious diseases, drugs, connective tissue diseases, and other extraneous diseases that were not well studied. I had a magnetic resonance angiogram (MRA) as well as invasive procedures like a full-brain angiogram (a procedure, done with some anesthesia, in which dye is injected from a huge catheter placed in a large blood vessel) and a transesophageal echocardiogram (TEE). A TEE is a sonographic procedure done under anesthesia in which a flexible endoscope is placed down the throat and into the upper portion of the gastrointestinal system, the esophagus. The esophagus sits behind the heart; therefore, an endoscope placed in the esophagus can give very good imaging of the nearby heart. The final findings revealed a patent foramen ovale (PFO): a small hole between the left and right atria of my heart. The doctors theorized that a small blood clot from the right atrium of my heart had crossed over to the left atrium (via the PFO) and subsequently into the blood vessels that take blood to my brain.

Next, I had to see a cardiothoracic surgeon to discuss repair of the PFO. When the surgeon came to visit me, he reviewed my history and explained that PFOs were very common in our population, but only very few people would develop any medical problems related to the PFO. He wanted me to have a bubble study, which was essentially a transthoracic echocardiogram (TTE)—a sonographic procedure in which the heart is viewed from a probe placed on the chest, rather than from a probe placed in the esophagus like in a TEE—with an agitated saline solution injected through an intravenous catheter placed in my vein. I was afraid to do the bubble study because the bubbles could move from the right side of my heart directly into my left side and then to my brain. Then I could have another stroke! However, I signed the consent form and underwent the bubble study, surviving without complications. The cardiothoracic surgeon looked at the results, which showed that the PFO was small, minimal bubbles having crossed from the right atrium to the left atrium. He said that it was not worth cracking my chest to repair a defect so small; therefore, after a week's worth of testing at Walter Reed, I was discharged with a history of stroke. The only thing wrong with me was a PFO that was not worth repairing. I returned to the sports medicine clinic the following week, having missed so much of the rotation.

At the end of the month, I flew back to Boston, but it was difficult to ignore everything that had just happened. I pondered my next step. Although I had a flutter of thoughts, I did not know where to start or what my future looked like. Afterward, I was contacted by a naval attorney; however, I do not remember much about the conversation, nor did I understand a lot of it at age twenty-three. Essentially, this attorney, who had been appointed to represent me, said that I could no longer be in the military and wanted to know what I wanted. I told her that I had had a stroke, but I had done nothing wrong. If I were discharged from the military, what would happen to my HPSP scholarship? I stated that it would be unfair to make me repay the previous three years of medical school since the stoke had not been my fault. She submitted my case, and I subsequently received an honorary discharge from the United States Navy. Even though I did not owe anything for the previous three years, I was now on my own. I then visited the financial department at BUSM and applied for a loan to finish school.

On the outside, I gave the world the impression that I was handling everything well. Even my roommate did not know what had occurred. On the inside, however, I was struggling with the diagnosis and what this meant for my future. What if it happened again? How could I have this PFO fixed and prevent another event? Perhaps the small iced coffee that I had drunk earlier that morning had put me in an arrhythmia that caused a blood clot to leave my heart and go to my brain, in spite of the fact that I had not had any chest pain, any jitteriness, or the feeling of a racing heart. I wondered whether I would be prone to more thromboembolic events (events related to blood clots) in the future. Another concern was what would happen if I needed orthopedic surgery and had to wear a cast for a long time. Or what if I had a baby? Pregnancy, in general, is a condition during which women are at an increased risk of thromboembolism (blood clots), but pregnancy in a woman with a significant thromboembolic event in her medical history could be life threatening. The thought of not having children made me extraordinarily depressed. I cried for many weeks. I struggled to decide whether I should have my tubes tied to avoid this problem. No, I did not need to have my tubes tied—abstinence was working so well. I was single. Admission into medical school and studying had been time consuming. There had been no time to meet a guy and get to know him well enough to marry him. I was only twenty-three years old. I still wanted to live a long, productive life. I was too young and, at that time, not aware of the many options related to having a baby. Having a baby was also not a priority at that age. First, I needed to consider my own survival. After many weeks of deliberation, I finally concluded that I needed to just worry about today and try to finish medical school. Then I started to count my blessings. I'd had a stroke, but I had recovered 100 percent of all function. I did not owe thousands of dollars for my first three years of medical school. I needed to do what I had always done: figure out how to survive today and figure out tomorrow when it arrived.

I was lucky that most of my evaluation had been done at Walter Reed, which meant I did not have any medical bills. The only thing that I paid for out of pocket was the MRI that I'd had at the outpatient facility prior to my admission to Walter Reed, which cost me $1,000! The radiology unit did not send the bill to me, probably because they did not have my home address—I'd been sent over from the sports medicine clinic in Annapolis. So, they sent my name to a collection agency. The first time that I knew I had a bill was when the collection agency looked up my address and sent it! It is terrible what patients go through; it is difficult enough being a patient and dealing with the uncertainty of your own mortality, but having to deal with the financial aspect, especially as a poor student, made my medical condition even more unbearable. This was my first introduction to medical debt, a crisis faced by many Americans.

Even though a few weeks had passed, I was not ready to speak with anyone regarding my emotions after the stroke. However, I wanted help from a father or mother figure. My parents are amazing, but they could not help me with this, so I made an appointment with an OB-GYN doctor, Dr. Edelin, who I admired academically and who had taught me so much. Several times on Thanksgiving, he'd invited students who did not have a place to go to for the holiday to spend it at his house, so I'd gotten to see a personal side of him as well. I told him the entire story; he was glad that I was fine, but I needed follow-up care with a doctor in Boston. He found an amazing neurologist at Massachusetts General Hospital (MGH) who specialized in strokes. I will forever be grateful for everything that my colleague did for me. Dr. Edelin was one of the many mentors who shaped my life, watching me grow from an unassuming island kid to a competent physician. I confided to him my fears, including what I'd been going through since the stroke.

A pioneer in his field, Dr. Edelin fought for patient rights. Before *Roe v. Wade*, women had sought abortions from nonphysician providers, and some women had used hangers to induce their abortions at home. These women then showed up to the hospital with infected uteri. Some of them lost their reproductive organs in order to get rid of the infection; sadly, many of them lost their lives. Although this courageous doctor had been found guilty of manslaughter after performing a safe and lawful abortion in 1973, his conviction was later overturned. He championed the women who had no voice and triumphed when faced with so much adversity in his time. This amazingly accomplished physician gave me advice even after medical school. Unfortunately, Dr. Edelin died of cancer several years ago. The world lost a legend, and I lost a mentor and father figure. I am thankful that he enriched my life. Boston Medical Center dedicated a public square in his memory in 2017.

Following our talk, I made an appointment with the neurologist at MGH, which I had heard so much about. The legendary MGH was well known for patient excellence and is the original and largest teaching hospital of Harvard Medical School. Many amazing research studies have been done there. I met with the neurologist and reviewed all the details of my stroke. Many months had gone by, and he was glad that I had recovered 100 percent. Similar to what I'd been told at Walter Reed, this neurologist was not sure if I would have another stroke; however, he did promise to discuss my case at grand rounds and several interdepartmental meetings. A grand round is a large meeting of physicians in which they discuss difficult and interesting medical cases, which allows several doctors to give their opinions and to formulate a viable medical plan for the patient(s) under consideration. My case was so interesting and unusual that it would be presented at multiple physician meetings. I was not thrilled about being a medical mystery; I just wanted an answer to my problem.

Many months went by. I had continued with my original plan to split my fourth year of medical school into two years so I could do international work. With the help of several physicians, I had organized a three-month trip to Mexico. The neurologist called me a few weeks before I left for Mexico and told me that he could not guarantee that another stroke would not happen. Now that I would be outside the country, he was very worried. Although he did not say it, I knew he did not think it was safe for me to travel internationally for such an extended time. It had been six months since my stroke, and I felt healthy and normal, so I decided that I was not going to live in fear; I went ahead with the trip. My parents were not happy with my decision either.

It turns out that going to Mexico was what I really needed to do, because I not only gained a lot of medical experience but, more importantly, grew emotionally. The trip was a "great breath of fresh air" that really got my mind off my problems and onto trying to help others with their problems. I had completely let go of everything I left behind in Boston.

When I arrived in Mexico City, the designated guide took me to the home where I would stay for three months. It was the home of a single mother whose adult son lived with her. There were several bedrooms in the unit; I had a bedroom with an attached bathroom for my personal use. Even though I paid rent and bought my own food to put in the fridge, this woman was unbelievably kind to me and treated me like a daughter. She always invited me to go out with her and her friends, and I enjoyed their company. I practiced my Spanish with them and learned a lot about their culture. Her son spoke English, so when I got frustrated with speaking Spanish, I spoke to him in English, as he was always happy to practice his English skills. She guided me on where to find the bus, subway, local grocery store, and bakery.

The first of the three months in Mexico, I worked with an international expert on pediatric infectious diseases. I participated in a project evaluating the effects of vitamin A and zinc supplements on diarrhea in children living in rural areas of Mexico, diarrhea being, coincidentally, the same thing that Nikki had died of many years before. One of the nurses and I took the subway and buses to various rural parts of Mexico daily to study vitamin supplementation and infectious diarrhea. Initially, the subway was intimidating, so I was lucky to have her educate me on how to use it. We called the buses "chicken buses"—there were people aboard literally selling fruits, vegetables, and livestock from off the farm. Our study sites were small, rural towns where access to any medical care was very poor. When we arrived, we usually went to the local clinical locations where vitamin-enriched fluids were stored. From there, we loaded up our bags with the fluids and made our way to the nearby villages on foot. My colleague kept detailed notes about which children were assigned to which vitamins and asked their parents about gastrointestinal symptoms. These families were unbelievably poor; many lived in small homes made of mud or clay, and only a few had electricity. However, they always had kind personalities, and the children were always happy. My friend had developed such a good relationship with everyone since she visited the villages frequently.

The following two months in Mexico, I worked at the Gea González Hospital doing obstetrics and gynecology. This was a very busy hospital with approximately thirty deliveries per day, so I learned how to deliver babies and repair episiotomies (small vaginal cuts made to increase the space for a baby to deliver vaginally). The resident physicians taught me a lot, and once my obstetric skills were good, they let me do all the easy deliveries and participate in cesarean sections. The patients were grateful for my help, and I was truly grateful to be part of one of the best moments of their lives.

The physicians also allowed me to participate in gynecologic surgeries such as hysterectomies. Many women came to the hospital with large, painful fibroids in their uteri and bleeding that required hysterectomies. Because access to medical care was limited in that part of Mexico, these women came in only when the symptoms were unbearable. Hence, removal of large fibroid uteri was very common.

I was very busy for all three months but had every weekend free, so I used the weekends to see the highlights of Mexico: the National Museum of Anthropology, the National Museum of Art, the Basílica de Santa María de Guadalupe, the Frida Kahlo Museum, the murals of Diego Rivera, Chapultepec Castle, Paseo de la Reforma, the Centro Histórico, the Museo del Templo Mayor, and the Palacio de Bellas Artes. Then I travelled to various other parts of Mexico, including San Miguel de Allende, Coyoacán, Teotihuacán, Puebla, Guanajuato, Veracruz, and Guadalajara. I figured out how to take tour buses, although I got lost several times and had to ask the locals for directions. On the bright side, my Spanish improved even more. The more I travelled, the more enriched my life became.

In May 2001, I returned to Boston in time to see my classmates graduate. I was excited to see them move on to the next step, and I had no regrets about my decision to split my last year into two years. Already, I felt that I had grown in many more dynamic ways than I could possibly explain. Several months later, I made a follow-up appointment with the neurologist, who then referred me to a cardiologist and an interventional cardiologist. I met with a physician at Massachusetts General Hospital who had an amazing reputation but was still incredibly nice and social. He had been using catheterization—a minimally invasive way to close interatrial heart defects—and we explored the possibility of using it to treat my PFO, the only abnormality found on my extensive workup. If the PFO had been the true cause of my stroke, then the procedure would completely prevent me from having another one. After he explained the risks, benefits, indications, alternatives, success, and limitations of the procedure, I signed the informed consent form.

I'd stayed a full week at Walter Reed for the extensive evaluation, but I had not had any surgeries up until this point. The day of my procedure, I arrived at MGH having had nothing to eat after midnight, checked in, and changed into my hospital gown. My sister came with me. I was doing well until they wheeled me into the procedure room and asked me to move from the stretcher to the procedure table. I had anxiety written all over my face. A very nice nurse comforted me so I could receive general anesthesia for the procedure. The next thing that I remembered was waking up in the recovery room with a heavy ice pack on my sore right groin. Although the procedure had gone well, they were going to keep me overnight on cardiac monitoring. My throat was tender from intubation (the use of a breathing tube during my procedure), and I was not allowed to walk for several hours, until I had formed a clot in my right femoral vessel. I recall the first time I was able to get up and use the restroom, which was such a relief since I had tried the bedpan but been too embarrassed to make proper use of it. I have since had several follow-up bubble study echocardiograms, which were all normal. I had the PFO closed without having open-heart surgery. Thankfully, today, I can wear nice blouses without being embarrassed about a large scar on my chest!

As a child, I had always been fascinated by my fingernail beds. Since we lived in a tropical climate where the temperature was always in the eighties or nineties in degrees Fahrenheit, I'd never had cold fingers, yet my fingernail beds were blue whereas my sisters' were pink. Amazingly, after my heart surgery, my beds turned pink—problem solved.

Even though I did not know it back then, my stroke changed my life. Before my stroke, I had been a smart kid who had seen loss in both her personal and professional life. After my stroke, however, I'd had the opportunity to walk in the shoes of a patient. I now knew what it was like to be poked and prodded, to have catheters placed in various orifices, arteries, and veins, and to sit in a cardiac unit on a monitor and listen to the alarm sound off every few hours, with nurses coming in to see how I was doing. Furthermore, before my stroke, I'd seen the world in black and white. Now, I saw the world in a million shades of gray. Before, I'd wanted to keep pushing myself academically as much as possible, but now, although I am still self-driven, I always make time to smell the roses. There is something to be said for approaching your own morbidity and mortality and being given a second chance at "normal" life. I can now say that I personally understand the uncertainty of human existence. Each morning that I rise, I continue to thank God that I am alive and healthy to see the dawn of another day.

Fourteen

Residency

I am very lucky to have gone to medical school in Boston, to have met outstanding physicians, and to have been attended to by such caring doctors. Although I was very happy there, I struggled through six winters, which was a lot for a person who'd grown up in the Virgin Islands. I did not have depression in the winter, but I possibly had mild seasonal affective disorder. Every June, I was elated for the arrival of the sun and warm weather. I had so much energy during this time, but this energy only endured for three months. Unfortunately, I did not feel the weather warming up in March with the start of spring; instead, I felt it in June. I clearly needed much warmer weather to function.

As a result, I did not apply for residency in Boston but started looking south. I knew that my advisors were disappointed in me for not staying, but I needed a break from the bitter cold. The school still awarded me the David Rothbaum, MD, Award, which is given to the medical student who exhibited the most assertion in the obstetrics and gynecology third-year clerkship. I am forever thankful for the education I received at BUSM.

I did, however, enjoy my residency interviews. It was fun visiting other schools and learning about their curricula. The residency match process is a lottery in which students rank the residency programs and residency programs rank the students. Then the computer matches up the wish lists via an algorithm. Typically, the match happens in the spring, but the military match is a few months earlier. Hence, my sister knew that she would be moving to join the naval program in San Diego several months before I knew where I would attend residency. The local news came to BUSM's match day, and I just happened to be in the right place at the right time, because one of the school officials asked whether the news crew could document me opening my match envelope. They attached a microphone box to my clothes and filmed the event, during which all the students gather in the mail room for the big reveal of their matches. As we all opened our envelopes together, there was an abundance of excitement. I opened my envelope; I would be moving to Houston. Later that evening, my sister and I watched the news and witnessed my few seconds of fame.

My sister and I sold the few furniture items that we had in Boston, packed our books and clothes, and moved, she to San Diego and I to Houston. My dad helped me for a few weeks until I was settled into an apartment I had found in one of the many complexes near the Astrodome; it was an area where a mass of students and health-care professionals lived. I moved into a clean one-bedroom unit on the first floor. However, after a couple of days, I broke out into hives, although my dad did not. I am allergic to cats and dogs, and it turned out that the previous tenant had probably had pets. After lots of Benadryl and steroid creams—and another cleaning of the carpet—my hives improved.

I was anxious to start my residency. Since I am a student at heart, exploring more about medicine brought me an abundance of excitement. Also, I could not wait to absorb all the data in my new textbooks. Unfortunately, all that enthusiasm was curtailed by a poor working environment. We worked as much as 120 hours per week with shifts as long as 40 hours. That kind of schedule brought out the worst in people. As fast as you could check one item off your list of things to do, twenty more appeared. What kept me going were the patients, most of whom were grateful for someone to listen and take care of them.

Life was very difficult during residency. Several residents got divorced during this time frame, and I certainly did not have time to date. We were always exhausted; I remember several events that speak to how tired I was during that time. I was in the prime of my life (my mid to late twenties) and in excellent health, but my health was not enough for what I had to endure. One morning, I drove home after working a very long shift. I was almost there when I exited the freeway and stopped at a red light. It was the first time my body had stopped moving in over forty hours. Suddenly, I heard a thump. I had briefly fallen asleep, and my foot had come off the brake, which resulted in my car gently tapping the one in front of me. A very nice man came out of the car, where his family was waiting. He asked me if I was fine, and I admitted that it was my fault and I was sorry. We both evaluated the cars for damage; there was no damage to either car, so we shook hands and drove off. That happened in the first few months of my intern year, which is the first year of residency. Ever since then, I have always had the radio blasting with loud music, chewed gum, and/or talked on speakerphone on my drive home; it was the only way to stay awake.

During my residency, I enjoyed cooking even though I had very little time to do so. I decided to cook on the weekends and pack food in Tupperware to keep in the fridge and eat during the week. One weekend, I worked excessively and did not have the time or energy to cook, so during that week, I had to cook when I came home on the weekdays. I decided to buy items that I could cook in twenty minutes or less. One night, I came home and started cooking; the meal still had another ten to fifteen minutes to simmer down, so I figured I had enough time to take a quick shower. Wrong. The next thing I knew, the smoke detector alarm was sounding off. I jumped out of the shower, ran to the stove, and looked at the clock. It was fifteen minutes later. I couldn't believe that fifteen minutes had gone by so quickly; I had fallen asleep standing in the shower!

Because we were so busy during residency, we had very little time to take care of things like calling the phone company when there was a problem. I had all three services (phone, internet, and television) bundled, but there was a problem with my bill. I called the company one evening after I came home from work, and they put me on hold. I am not sure how long I was on hold, but I fell asleep on the couch and dropped the phone on the ground. When I finally woke up, I had to redial. Back in those days, I still paid my bills by postal mail; one night, I finally went through all my mail and bills for the month and discovered that, somehow, I'd mailed the payment for the utilities bill to the phone company and the payment for the phone bill to the utilities company. Oops.

Time continued to be a commodity in residency. One winter, I suffered from a sore throat, cough, sputum production, and low-grade fevers for over a month. I was tested for strep throat and pneumonia, but both tests were negative; I had only a common cold. If I could have slept it off, I would have been better in just a few days, but with the long hours of work, my body and immune system were struggling despite my youth. Another health problem was discovered during my second year of residency in my routine annual exam with my gynecologist. Given my past medical history,

I always try to see a doctor instead of having one of my colleagues write a script. The exam discovered a breast lump. Wonderful—just my luck! I had a breast sonogram and a mammogram. The breast sonogram showed two small masses, smaller than one centimeter, in my right breast, so I needed a biopsy. Luckily, my night float rotation was coming up, which meant I worked at nights but had the days free. I was always exhausted and needed the days to sleep, but the timing of this rotation worked out well: I could go for my breast biopsy one morning after work. Since I did not need anesthesia for the biopsy, I could drive there myself.

I had an ultrasound-guided stereotactic biopsy that day. They needed to take several samples, so a very large needle pierced my breast nine times to get a sample of sufficient quantity from both lesions. I am glad I have good pain tolerance—it was more painful than anticipated. The next couple of weeks were stressful as I waited for the biopsy results. If I had cancer, what would that mean for the rest of my career? For my life? Had they caught it at an early stage, where there would be an excellent prognosis? Although I do not have a family history of breast cancer, many patients with breast cancer do not. I did have other risk factors, including being at a young age during my first menses, ovulating every month, never using birth control, and never being pregnant. My gynecologist made a referral for me to see a breast surgeon. I was sure that I had cancer, but really, the gynecologist just wanted a breast surgeon to look over my case. Thankfully, the biopsy results were negative for breast cancer. I finally exhaled.

As part of my residency training, I had to rotate as a physician on the women's ward in the local jail. I remember the horrified feeling I had the first time that I walked into the building; I had never stepped into a jail until then. Visitors had to go through the metal detector and several locked iron gates. There were women there who were pregnant and/or had sexually transmitted infections; most did not have custody of their children, and they needed care too. It was not my role to judge them; they had already been judged by a dozen of their peers. I had empathy toward these women because many had had amazingly hard lives that had led them to their current situation. The jail rotation was incredibly difficult for me emotionally.

In the fall of my intern year, I rotated through the reproductive endocrinology and infertility (REI) department. I absolutely fell in love with this subspecialty. A woman's ability to conceive can be both a joyous and terrifying time in her life. As many as one in eight women had problems conceiving and really needed help, yet only a small portion would seek out that help. The joy on their faces when they finally conceived was invaluable. Now that I had identified what I wanted to do with my life, the next step was how to get there. REI is an unbelievably competitive field since so few people are selected. I needed to make myself a competitive and attractive candidate, so I sought out the help of two people. One of the REI doctors at the university conducted a lot of research in addition to seeing patients. To get into an REI fellowship, I needed a fair amount of solid research under my belt, so I made an appointment with him to see if I could participate in one of his projects. He was extraordinarily kind to me and took me under his wing. Unfortunately, he already had a full-time employee dedicated to doing the bench research, so I was not a help to him. If anything, I was a hindrance! They had to stop to teach me basic science research. The good news is that I was highly self-motivated and learned quickly. I came into the lab on the weekends and many days after nightly call to keep my project going; in my second year of residency, I even used one of my vacation weeks to finish, completing the project one year earlier than anticipated. I presented my project at the end of my second year of residency and won first prize. That was a rewarding feeling; I had made lots of sacrifices and invested many hours of my free time toward it.

The work, however, was not yet done: I also needed clinical experience. The second person who helped me was an REI physician in a practice affiliated with the university. He taught me many clinical "pearls" and encouraged me to write case reports of some of our interesting findings, which were later presented as posters at the American Society for Reproductive Medicine (ASRM). In addition, he invited me to come to his private clinic to observe an egg retrieval. Since this dedicated doctor did some of the REI surgeries at the university, I was excited to be able to attend his surgical cases. I had a hunger for more knowledge and am still friends with him today. Once I became a practicing physician, my new colleague insisted that I call him by his first name, but it took a long time before I was comfortable doing that. Now, we have an outstanding collegial relationship.

I applied for an REI fellowship in the fall of 2005. The four years of my obstetrics/gynecology residency were not enough, so I needed to do a three-year fellowship in REI to eventually practice fertility. I applied to several programs and went on a series of interviews. Once again, I used my vacation days to further my career by scheduling my interviews then. I felt that all the interviews went well, but the programs across the country jointly received hundreds of applications for only a few spots.

Match day came around. At match hour (twelve o'clock noon), I had to log in to the match website to find out if I had been chosen. There was no shortage of work in residency, though, and it was well past noon by the time I finished a cesarean section. Instead of trying to find lunch, I had to find an available computer to log on. My profile said that I'd matched to the New Jersey Medical School (NJMS) program. Although I was happy, I was still in shock. The fellowship process was extraordinarily competitive that year. I closed the browser and logged in again just to be sure; the same thing came up. I was going to move to New Jersey in the summer of 2006 to start my training in REI.

Fifteen

The Fellowship Years: A Reminder That I Cannot Take My Health for Granted

I moved to New Jersey in June 2006. Finding an apartment was difficult. I had made a trip up to New Jersey earlier but had not been able to find an affordable apartment in a safe neighborhood; I returned to Texas unsuccessful. The school was located in Newark, which had a history of high crime. Byron, the nephew of one of my mother's friends, helped me. I did not know him at the time, but he lived in New Jersey and was the main reason I found a place to live. I had located a few apartments online, and since I could not make a second trip back up there, I asked him to go visit them to see whether they were habitable. I did not know New Jersey at all and was not sure which towns were safe. An apartment I sent him to visit in Nutley turned out to be perfect for me.

There, I moved into a second-floor apartment. One of the neighbors on the first floor was a sweet lady in her eighties, a typical Italian grandmother who introduced herself as Sofia. She had several children and grandchildren, all of whom were involved in her life. Her husband had passed away when she was just in her fifties, so she had been single since then. Sofia was full of spark and independence. She gave me tips on where to go for groceries, the gym, and the pharmacy and on how to take public transportation to New York City when I wanted to be a tourist. She became a close neighbor and friend, and I am still in contact with her today. This kind soul was yet another angel who took me under her wings.

For me, fellowship hours were much better than residency. The first year included only bench research projects in the laboratory and writing scientific documents. I planned my days around the experiments. While my samples were running on the machine, I had time to review articles to improve my research. By the end of my fellowship, I had read, in detail, over one hundred articles and how they pertained to my project and, ultimately, my thesis. I knew my thesis material inside and out. My advisor grilled me regularly on it—and, yes, she was very tough on me. But I credit her for my ability to now read and write scientific articles amazingly well. My second year of fellowship—my favorite year—was all clinical. I really enjoyed the hands-on work of taking care of patients. My fellowship program director was a positive role model; I learned so much from him. To this day, I continue to look to him for advice. The third year of fellowship involved a few clinical rotations in medical and pediatric endocrinology as well as finishing my thesis.

During the first year of my fellowship, I turned thirty. I had spent my teen years in high school and college trying to figure out how to get into medical school; I had spent the first half of my twenties in medical school and the second half in residency. Consequently, I'd never had time for my personal life. Things were now a bit easier, and, for the first time, I had free time. Turning thirty was a wake-up call. I needed to meet someone, hopefully get married, and work on having children, so I tried Match.com. I went on some terrible dates that are not even worth mentioning. Additionally, I went on several speed-dating events, at which I met three different guys.

The first guy and I had a natural connection. He was educated and handsome, had a great sense of humor, and worked in Manhattan. We exchanged information and photos. No, I did not send any naughty selfies—just photos so that we could look at each other regularly. We also started having phone conversations. During the third conversation, he mentioned that he had to go home to Romania to take care of some business and finalize his divorce. He then proceeded to tell me about all the business in Romania that he needed to take care of. The very next thing that came out of my mouth was, "So you are still legally married?" Dating a married man or someone recently divorced and finding his way was not an ideal situation. I thought it was clever of him to just slip that into the conversation. He got it off his chest and made me aware but did not give any explanation until I asked further. We never made it to our first date. The second guy was kind, respectable, and also a physician. There was, however, no spark. We would make great colleagues and friends but nothing more. The third guy I had lunch with. Although he never outright said so, it became clear that he had lied about his age and was not looking for anything long term. I did not call him after the first date.

I tried eHarmony next, signing up for three months. I connected with Ron in my first three days, although he had been on the website for quite some time. We met for coffee on a Sunday. He was a handsome man with a quiet demeanor and a dry sense of humor. He had graduated from Princeton and was now working as a software architect. That day, we talked for an hour, just enough for a typical first date; the date went well. I knew I wanted to see him again, and vice versa. He called me several times after the date.

Three days after our first date, on a brisk January evening, I took New Jersey Transit into New York City for a monthly obstetrics/gynecology meeting. On the ride home, it started to snow. I had parked my car at the train station, which was maybe a five-minute drive from my apartment. When I got off the train, I missed the gap to the landing, stepped out with my right foot, and slipped on the wet snow. Even with the noisy train in the background, I heard a loud pop. I knew something bad had happened. As an athletic person, I compensated extremely well. I got up and walked to my car, cleaned the snow from my windshield, and drove off. My ankle never felt right after that incident; it did not feel stable enough to hold me up. So, I bought an ankle brace from a foot store, hoping that if I wore it for a few weeks, I would be better. Since I walked fine with the soft ankle brace in my shoe, no one ever really knew what I was going through. But I never got better. Several weeks later, I saw my primary care doctor, who ordered an X-ray. It did not show any broken bones, so he had me go see a physical therapist for a possible sprain. I spent the next year and nine months seeing five different physical therapists, three orthopedic surgeons, and one physical medicine and rehabilitation doctor. Additionally, I received steroid shots in my ankle, without any relief. The muscles in my foot compensated well, and I also have excellent pain tolerance—certainly, I have never been described as a complainer—so I carried out my everyday functions easily; however, these compensations worked against me. Even though I looked and walked fine with my brace, something was structurally wrong with my ankle. But no one else was seeing it.

The fifth physical therapist was another angel God placed in my path. She got me as healthy as possible, but once we got to a certain stage in my progress, I could not go further. In fact, I deteriorated. She told me what I'd kept telling doctors: something was wrong with the structure of my ankle. I saw an orthopedic surgeon in New Jersey, who was very rude; nevertheless, he at least ordered an MRI, something that had not been done in all this time. I got a copy of the

MRI images and took them to a doctor at the Hospital for Special Surgery in New York City. After listening to my complaints, he took a look at the MRI images and confirmed that many of the ligaments in my ankle were torn. What was seen on my MRI was scar tissue, not functional ligaments. That was why I could not recover well; scar tissue does not function like a ligament. He needed to take a tendon from another part of my body and then use this as a graft to replace the ligaments that had been torn. I would then have to do a lot of physical therapy after the surgery.

Ron and I continued to date during this time. We went to Niagara Falls; Woods Hole and Provincetown in Massachusetts; Wildwood and Atlantic City in New Jersey; and California twice, along with numerous weekend adventures to the local zoo, theaters, wine tastings, and botanical gardens. Every free moment was spent on an adventure. As long as I had a brace in my shoe, I could walk for miles, so my ankle never affected our relationship. His mom, who had three sons, loved me. The two younger sons were extroverts, were married, and had children. Ron, her eldest son, was an introvert. Although she never said so, it was clear that Ron was her favorite. He looked exactly like her. She was happy that he might be settling down. As a result, she was unbelievably kind to me and would have been an excellent mother-in-law. Ron was almost seven years older than me, as well as an amazing, kind, wonderful person. Although I had been on dates in the past, he was my first relationship. In the past, he had been in a long-term relationship for many years, but it had not worked out. Both he and I were great people; we were just not right together. I was and still am a very happy person, but it was my first relationship, and I was too scared back then to address the elephant in the room. Things never felt easy, but I thought that is what you were supposed to do: try to make things work. Maybe I did not want to start all over again on the dating scene, so I tried hard to make things work in my current relationship. Back then, whenever we got into a disagreement, we would find something fun for us to talk about or do so we could get past the conflict. In reality, the unresolved disagreement was still there, just swept under the rug.

In many ways, though, Ron was another angel that God sent to me. I found a friend and travel buddy in him, and we had so many fun adventures together. He was also there for my ankle surgery. He took me to the hospital for my procedure, which took longer than anticipated. I had more scar tissue than was imaginable, and a large nerve was injured during the surgery. I stayed with Ron afterward, thinking that I would be able to move back into my apartment after a few weeks. But my recovery was long; instead of moving back to my apartment after two weeks, it took six. I still, however, had a long road to recovery ahead of me. During this time, I started to drive myself even though it was my right leg that was damaged. I drove using my knee joint since I did not have any range of motion in my ankle joint. In this way, I figured out how to compensate and be self-sufficient. It was not easy, but I did what I'd always done and found a way to survive.

Meanwhile, Ron had met my parents, and they liked him. He even came to St. Croix that winter for Christmas; I was hoping that the vacation trip would fix things for us. We got to our two-year dating anniversary, but things had been rocky since the first anniversary. I had learned a lot during the past year, but it was now clear that we should go separate paths. I was going to graduate from fellowship in six months, and I had already contracted with a job in New Jersey following my fellowship. Even though I did not like the cold weather, I'd chosen to stay in New Jersey so I could be close to Ron and his family. But it was not enough. We broke up and got back together numerous times after our two-year anniversary. However, in the end, I cut it clean: I stopped responding to calls, texts, and emails. We had more than given our relationship a fair shot.

Unlike my stroke, after which I regained 100 percent of neurologic function by the third day, I struggled for two years after the ankle surgery before I sensed a complete return to function. Four months after the surgery, the injured nerve in my right foot awoke. Because of the injured nerve, I'd had no sensation or movement in the ankle, which had severely impaired my recovery. Once my nerve woke up, my physical therapy became effective. The injury, surgery, and recuperation left me once again handicapped. My primary care doctor at that time wrote a note so I could have a disability tag in my car for three to six months. Always a strong-willed person, I had usually parked at the far end in parking lots so I could have an excuse to walk some distance and get some exercise. Now, I was disabled and could barely walk a few steps. I so wanted to be healthy again. Being healthy and walking from the back of the parking lot to the store was much better than being disabled and parking right in front of the store.

Unfortunately, I had to learn to walk again. I'd thought that after learning this as a baby, I would never have to learn again. Wrong. Like a baby, I started off by standing on two legs and holding both crutches. Then I let go of one crutch; then I let go of both crutches but stood next to a wall just in case I needed to hold on to something to prevent a fall. I then practiced putting one foot in front of the other. I also had to work on various rubber-band exercises that moved my ankle in countless directions to increase the range of motion. My right leg was thinner than my left due to loss of muscle from lack of use. For a while, I walked with a boot and cane. Once there was more ankle function, I only needed a boot. Finally, I was able to let go of the cane. After ten months following the surgery, I could go up stairs easily; however, I could not reciprocate my legs— alternate them left and right—to come down stairs. Also, I was able to walk, but not over long distances or intensely without developing massive pain and swelling in my ankle. Reciprocation and longer walks both came later.

At this point, my insurance stopped paying for the remainder of my physical therapy. Once again, I was learning how difficult it is to be a patient. I was dealing with my physical condition, which was still not optimal; the emotional stress of going from a highly functioning, athletic woman to essentially a disabled person; and now the financial burden of how to do the rest of my therapy without insurance coverage. Was God really teaching me a second lesson? I had lived a life that I believed God would have approved of, and I already had been given a lot of life lessons to learn and grow from. Now, again, I was being reminded of my own morbidity and mortality. I really need to play the lottery with these odds!

With no insurance coverage, I had to come up with my own protocol. I was lucky to be a physician and very athletic, as my understanding of the human body was essential to developing my own therapy. First, I joined a fully functional gym. Since I was now working at my first job out of fellowship, I had a better income but less free time. The good news was that I was single. I did not have a spouse or children to worry about, so, in the evenings and on weekends, I worked on *me*. I developed a routine on the treadmill. I would run—more like walk very fast—for thirty seconds, then walk more slowly for thirty seconds. I did this for five minutes the first week, increased to six minutes the following week, then to seven, and so forth until I practiced this rotation for twenty minutes. This progression took about twenty weeks since there were some weeks when I was not able to advance another minute. I quickly learned that if I tried to take two steps forward instead of one, I would end up taking five steps back, so I had to push myself enough without overdoing it. Once I was able to do this for twenty minutes, I then adjusted the ratio—30 seconds of light running and 30 seconds of walking—from 30:30 to 35:25, then to 40:20, then 45:15, then 50:10, then 55:5, and finally 60:0. Now, I was able to do a light run / fast walk on the treadmill for twenty minutes straight. I then increased my speed by 0.1 miles per hour every three to four weeks until I got to a good running pace. I followed this strict regimen three times per week—Mondays, Wednesdays, and Fridays. Fridays were perfect for going to the gym because I did not have to wait for a treadmill. On the off days, I utilized the hot tub in the gym to loosen my muscles. Before I went to sleep every night, as well as upon awakening every morning, I placed an ice pack around my right ankle for twenty minutes to decrease the swelling. Thankfully, I completed my ankle recovery protocol two years after the surgery.

Unfortunately, due to my right ankle's limitations, I'd developed compensatory left piriformis syndrome. Essentially, for several years, I had subconsciously put the majority of my body weight on my left leg to guard my right ankle, which led to all the muscles in my left leg tightening up to hold me upright. The tight muscles became spastic and caused compression of the sciatic nerve running down my left leg, which led to severe sciatic pain even though I had no back or disc problems. Today, I still struggle with occasional flares of pain related to piriformis syndrome.

Sixteen

Emotional and Physical Recovery

At the gym in South Jersey where I performed my ankle recovery protocol, there was a weekly Sunday ballroom class. I now lived in the suburbs, and having not danced since high school, I figured that I would go to the class. The class was very small, but our instructor was full of life and enthusiasm. I also met two other students, a couple who, like myself, always arrived fifteen minutes or more before the class started. Therefore, I had ample opportunity to get to know them. Joann was eighty-seven years old at that time, and Walt was just slightly older than her. Avid dancers when they were young, they both downplayed their dancing skills quite a bit. It was clear the first time I saw them dancing together that they had done this before. Joann was so light on her feet. The instructor taught us the basics of the waltz, foxtrot, East Coast and West Coast swing, rumba, salsa, merengue, and cha-cha. We had so much fun. Since I was still in the process of finishing my ankle recovery regimen, this easier pace of dancing was fun. More importantly, I gained from this class a handful of extremely sincere friends with whom I am still in contact today.

Our instructor's energy was addictive. Once we were all good at dancing, she arranged various gigs at local restaurants where we could go and dance. Sometimes, she did the singing. She introduced me to a woman named Beth, who was also an amazing dancer. Beth lived in Philadelphia; she and I were in the same age range and were both single. Beth quickly became my buddy for dance socials. On Sunday nights, I had been going to Dance Haddonfield by myself because it was well organized and so much fun. Many of the attendees were much older but were exceptional dancers. There was a class for one hour, and then the social dancing started. Most of the dancers would rotate, so even though I did not show up with a partner, I was always able to dance a few songs.

Joann became one of my best friends; today, I consider her my second mother. She is another angel sent to me by God. Joann invited me to her house for Thanksgiving, Easter, and practically every holiday that I could not go home to see my parents. I looked through her albums during one of my visits to her house. She was immensely beautiful in her wedding pictures; Joann and Walt were a beautiful couple both on the outside and on the inside, and the love that they shared was fascinating. They had gotten married in their early twenties and were close to their seventieth anniversary when I met them. Walt still looked at Joann with unbelievably loving eyes. I had known them for about a year and a half when Walt passed away. Joann was heartbroken; she had known Walt for most of her entire life. They had a love that transcended all time, but they also worked very hard at their relationship. They'd had difficult times, which Joann told me many stories of, but their love was stronger than any obstacle thrown their way. Together, they raised three amazing, successful children, along with grandchildren and great-grandchildren.

Joann was another typical Italian grandmother, and I enjoyed cooking with her. She made all meals from scratch, even her pasta, starting with flour and churning out pasta shapes. Joann took care of me like I was her daughter. One day, after I'd struggled for a year with bloody stools, she took me to the hospital for my colonoscopy. It turned out that I just had internal hemorrhoids; however, she insisted that I stay with her following my procedure. She gave me a pair of warm, fuzzy blue socks to wear for my colonoscopy. Since then, I have worn those socks for every procedure that I have had, including my egg retrievals. In her late eighties and early nineties, she still drove—long distances, too, including visiting her daughter, Diann, in Maryland. Because Joann had hip problems in her early nineties and had repair surgery, she has had intermittent hip pain for years. Now, she only drives on the local roads to the grocery store. Diann is like a sister to me, and I have spent many holidays at her Maryland home. Diann even visited my house in Texas on one of her business trips. Her daughter, Julie, is a beautiful, smart, talented young woman who was a competitive swimmer for quite some time. Julie crocheted an extraordinary blanket for our Leo; we brought Leo home from the hospital wrapped in that blanket. There are no words that completely describe how lucky I am to have Joann in my life. I love her immeasurably.

Not surprisingly, dancing continued to open my social circle. I started taking salsa and bachata classes at the Atrium, a dance studio in South Jersey. The dance classes were always filled, a testament to how good the owner/instructor was. Under her tutelage, my Latin dancing improved dramatically, and I now feel comfortable walking out onto a dance floor anytime there is a Latin song playing. This amazing dancer held dance parties on Saturday nights twice monthly at the Atrium. Initially, I was nervous about going to a dance party where I knew there were more skillful dancers. But, after a few parties, I had gained enough confidence to make this a regular routine.

I found many friends at the Atrium, many of whom invited me to other dance events. Alma, an unbelievably beautiful woman from Guatemala, and I started classes there together, and we quickly became close friends. We shopped, dined, and attended dance events together. One December, just before Christmas, we took a tour bus to Hershey, Pennsylvania, where we took a fantastic tour of Hershey's chocolate factory. It was magical; I was a kid in a chocolate candy world. Before heading back to South Jersey, the tour bus then drove us through Hershey Sweet Lights, two miles of wooded trails illuminated by almost six hundred animated displays. We marveled at the spectacular Christmas lights. It was truly a winter wonderland, and I felt like a child in an enchanted world. Alma and I still reminisce about that exquisite day.

I am always in awe at how things happen for a reason and how one event can open a new world. Had I not attended dance class at the gym, I would never have met all the amazing people that I have mentioned. All these people are still my friends; their friendship helped me get through my ankle recovery and the emotional recovery from my recent breakup with Ron. The people around me have influenced my life in so many positive ways.

Seventeen

Do I Voluntarily Become a Single Mother?

It was now several years since my stroke. My heart defect was closed, and my right ankle was functional. At one point while dating Ron, I'd considered getting pregnant by utilizing blood thinners during the pregnancy and postpartum periods. I would need blood thinners because of my past medical history of a stroke, even though my heart defect had been repaired. However, I was always unsure about my relationship with Ron and never brought up the topic of children. Besides, if I were to conceive with a man, I'd prefer marrying him first.

My right ankle was a bad reminder of what disability looked like. Pregnancy, even in and of itself, is associated with a higher risk of blood clots, and this risk is more elevated in a person who has already had one blood clot before—say, a person who has had a stroke. I made appointments with hematologists, cardiologists, and obstetricians, who all stated that they could not predict what would happen if I became physically pregnant. Surrogacy would be a safer option. The truth is I never went into the field of REI to help myself. I chose to become a doctor after feeling helpless when losing my sisters Nikki and Andromeda and my dear Granny. I chose obstetrics and gynecology because I wanted to help women. But then I fell in love with the subspecialty of REI because I wanted to give people the opportunity to have children. Until my fellowship, I worked only on my career. During my fellowship, I had hoped that things would work out with Ron, but they did not. I'd finished my studies and taken a job in New Jersey. It was during my first three years in private practice that I saw women using surrogates to become pregnant. One patient had a big influence on me; she was also of Indian descent, beautiful and smart but with a heart defect. She utilized a surrogate to have her baby. I figured I could do the same thing.

I worked in private practice in New Jersey for three years before deciding to move back to Texas. I had initially stayed in New Jersey to be closer to Ron, but since the relationship was over, there was no reason to stay there. Additionally, I was still not a fan of cold weather and snow. I was almost thirty-six years old when I moved to the Dallas–Fort Worth (DFW) area; I view everything in life as a new adventure. I'd loved living in Houston during residency; there was something about the warm weather and the amazing and energetic mood it put me in.

Right around my thirty-sixth birthday, the American Society for Reproductive Medicine (ASRM) came out and said that the benefits of egg freezing outweighed the risks. Egg freezing now opened the door for women to delay childbearing in order pursue other dreams or wait until they found the right partner. It is amazing how we work against women sometimes. We tell our female children to not get pregnant and to pursue their dreams. Then, suddenly, we switch the mantra to, "Why do you not have children?" Egg freezing was a way to bridge this gap.

I was older around the time of the ASRM announcement, and I wanted children more than anything. So, I froze a batch of eggs. Only four eggs were retrieved, but they were all of excellent quality for freezing. All women are different. Some have many eggs retrieved; some have few. Some of the eggs are of great quality; others are not. One thing is for sure: the more advanced the age, the lower the quantity and quality of the eggs.

While I had friends in Houston, Austin, and San Antonio, I did not know anyone in DFW. When I first arrived, I rented a small townhouse. I also wanted to grow my practice, so I went to various professional networking events in Dallas. One event was held at a wine room by a travel agency, which I figured would be an opportunity to meet people and also learn about various travel options, as I wanted to see the world. At the event, I met a nice woman. Although I had joined Meetup, I had not gone to any events. This woman and I talked extensively that night. She learned a lot about my interests and told me which Meetup groups to join. I went home for Christmas that winter to visit my parents but was in DFW for New Year's. I did not want to be alone on New Year's Eve, so I signed up for a Meetup New Year's dinner, which more than one hundred attended. The event started at 7:30 p.m. on New Year's Eve. I arrived early—a typical behavior for me. Though I am an extrovert and enjoy meeting new people, I sat in the parking lot, giving myself a pep talk because I was about to walk into a room where I did not know anyone. A small voice in my head said, "You could turn around now." But a louder voice said to just go in and see where it took me. In the end, I had so much fun that night. I made several key friends, all of whom invited me to other events that eventually opened up my social circle. That night, I was one of the last people to leave the New Year's party.

Now, with a solid social circle and an advancing age, I decided that it was time to settle into a home. I was self-sufficient, so I bought my first home. I also decided that being a mother was more important to me than ever before. Although I had not met the right soul mate, there were presently many women choosing to be single mothers. Utilization of donor sperm was quite common. I bought a home with enough room for one or two children and an extra bedroom for a nanny, a family member, or some other type of help—I could not do this all by myself.

When I started to look at agencies to find a surrogate, I discovered it was a much more difficult process than I had anticipated.

First, there are few women who want to do this. Then geography becomes an issue; I preferred someone in Texas. Besides these obstacles, there are multiple items that you need to match on with the surrogate, including concerns like what happens if there is something wrong with the baby and who decides. The surrogate, since she would be the one pregnant, would decide even though she would be carrying my baby. So, being aligned on many viewpoints was critical. I did a lot of soul searching before making the decision to be a single parent. Many of my friends were supportive of my decision, but a few worried about how I would be able to manage being a mother with everything else that I had going on in my life.

I found a wonderful surrogate through the agency. Since I have a medical background, I thought I knew what to look for. Wrong. There are many factors that affect who to pick as a surrogate. I chose a woman named Mandy because I did not have many options and I liked her profile. Mandy was a beautiful woman who was open to carrying for a single parent like myself. She already had two children of her own and did not want more children. Her medical background was clean, and she lived about two hours from me, so driving to appointments would have been easy. I met her and her fiancé at a local Panera Bread in their area. They were super nice; I hugged her the first time I met her. Surrogates are some of the most selfless people I have ever met, as they are willing to put themselves through the physical, mental, and emotional journey of pregnancy just to help another person become a parent. While they do receive a payment for this and have all their medical bills paid, it takes a special person to do such a magnificent thing for a stranger. Together, Mandy and I worked out the legal contracts easily and were ready to start.

To start the process, I decided to do another in vitro fertilization (IVF) cycle to get more eggs instead of thawing the four I had. I wanted to save those four eggs for a time when I was much older and could not produce any more eggs. Now I needed to find donor sperm. There are many credible sperm cryobanks in the country, and I looked at several. This was a time-consuming process: hair color, eye color, ethnic origin, education, and previous pregnancy success rates are just a few of the selective criteria. Despite the consumption of time, this was an important endeavor. I was choosing the other 50 percent of my child's (or children's) genetic makeup. On the cryobanks website, I made wish lists of my search criteria, which generated a list of donors that met the requirements. I then sat and read through each of these donor profiles. My favorite part of the process was reading the donors' short answers and essays regarding why they'd chosen to be donors. There were many truly altruistic people who just wanted to help another person who could not have children. Many of these donors spoke to me through the essays, and I gained a good sense of their personalities. After a long search, I finally settled on my donor. I ordered the sperm and had it shipped.

Because of my chosen profession, I was able to play a major role in this process. I organized and managed everything. One of my colleagues did the retrieval and transfer, something that I, as the patient, could not physically do. Six eggs were retrieved, and they were fertilized with donor sperm. Two embryos were transferred to Mandy. Her uterine lining was slow to thicken up, something I had not thought would happen in a woman who had conceived in the past. My embryos looked good under the microscope, but I had not done preimplantation genetic testing for aneuploidies (PGT-A). PGT-A evaluates embryos for their number of chromosomes or gene regions. We all have forty-six chromosomes—twenty-three pairs. One copy in each pair is inherited from the egg, the other copy from the sperm. The first twenty-two chromosomes are autosomes. The last pair—pair number twenty-three—are the sex chromosomes that determine gender. Euploid embryos have the right number of chromosomes or gene regions, but aneuploid embryos do not. Generally, euploids have a high chance of resulting in a baby.

I stayed positive the entire time, hoping that at least one embryo would take to the uterus. Mandy also stayed positive. She texted me several times, wondering if some symptoms that she was experiencing were pregnancy-related. It was too early to tell, as high levels of progesterone supplements (which she was taking) can make women have symptoms such as breast tenderness. The day of destiny rolled around: it was time for Mandy to have her serum pregnancy test. It turned out negative. All my staff knew and felt bad for me. I did what I always did: showed a proper, professional face and said, "There is still one more embryo frozen from this batch. We can try a frozen embryo transfer cycle in a few months." That day, I went home and had dinner. I spoke to Mandy and gave her hope; we would try again. Then I walked upstairs to the empty bedroom that I designated as the baby's room and cried uncontrollably.

Fortunately, I had one more embryo that could be used for a frozen embryo transfer (FET) cycle. An FET cycle involved having Mandy again take medications to make her uterus ready to receive the embryo; the embryo would then be thawed and transferred. We did the FET cycle a couple of months after the first transfer. This embryo was of good quality, though not as good as the first two, and no PGT-A testing was done. The pregnancy test was negative. Now I needed a mental and physical break. I was not ready to do this again. Mandy's pregnancy test came back negative on a Friday in October; after taking some time to think about it, I called the agency coordinator and Mandy on Saturday morning. Although I really liked her and enjoyed working with her, I needed to end our contract. Mandy was so understanding on the phone. I reminded her of how much she had done for me already but shared that I was not ready for another round. Perhaps I needed to think about just adopting or about having a very concrete plan if I wanted to do this again.

Many of my friends knew that I had intended to become a single mother, but only one friend knew that I had gone through with the process. In hindsight, I am glad I did not tell many people that I had gone through with it. There would have been too many concerned questions as to what was going on and why it was not working. My patients complain about this all too often. They want to tell family and friends about their fertility struggles; they need someone to talk to—many times just a sympathetic ear who will say, "Everything will be OK." Also, if family and friends know, then the patients will have the support they need both for when things go right and also for when things go wrong. But they do not want family and friends meddling, either. These patients do not want to always have to answer questions as to why things went wrong, what *they* will do next, and what *I* will do next.

In truth, I did not know what I wanted to do next. I just needed a break. I needed to pull my head out of the water and take a big breath before diving in again!

Eighteen

Meeting My Husband

The pregnancy test was negative on a Friday. The following Saturday, I had a Diwali lunch midday and a Halloween party to attend that evening. I was not on call but wanted to go to the office on Sunday for a couple of procedures, having promised several patients that I would do their procedures regardless of whether or not I was on call. The Diwali lunch was at an Indian restaurant in Irving. I am fourth generation-Indian, Pakistani, and Chinese. Although I attend a Christian church, my Indian friends always make an effort to invite me to their events. I could not find my sari that day, so I wore American clothes. One sari is all I have; my mom bought it for me on one of her trips home to Guyana. She thought I should have at least one Indian-cultured outfit. Even though Mom did not wear saris regularly, she always kept one for special Indian-cultured events. It turned out that there were a few people wearing American clothes to the Diwali lunch, so I did not feel singled out. It was very refreshing to go to lunch after having another negative pregnancy test. No one knew about my situation, and, therefore, I did not have to talk about it. I just had loads of fun. The lunch was buffet style. While I am a light eater, I did go back for seconds because the food was yummy. After lunch, we walked around Irving, shopping and burning off the calories. It was a beautiful October day, and the walk and social company were revitalizing. I quickly forgot about all my problems.

That evening, I attended the Halloween party, which was at the home of a woman named Linda. I had met her in January earlier that year, and we quickly bonded over salsa dancing. An astounding woman, she had volunteered at Oktoberfest a few weeks prior to her party. Her energy was addictive. I'd joined her and her friends at the end of her volunteer session at Oktoberfest, and we'd met several guys, one of whom was going to be at her Halloween party. He and I had connected at the festival; however, we never made it to our first date. The phone calls following Oktoberfest seemed odd. Although I had nothing against him, I did not want to have anything more than a brief conversation with him at the Halloween party. Earlier in the week, I had told one of my neighbors about him while debating whether or not to attend the Halloween celebration, and she'd reinforced what I felt. I really liked Linda, and I was going to her party because she was my friend and had invited me. It was the right thing to do. Besides, I wanted to go because Linda had told me how much time and energy she had put into preparing for it.

This was my first time visiting Linda's home, which had the best Halloween decorations I had ever seen. The front yard had giant, inflatable monsters, and there were tombstones in the yard with hands coming out of the ground to mimic the rising dead. Inside, the entire place was fully decorated. She had cobwebs, spooky pictures that looked back at you and mimicked your movement, skeletons, and monsters in every corner. Linda had a full bar with a bartender that she'd hired for the night. He made fantastic cocktails, according to the other attendees, and he had funny names for his drinks, like "blood of the vampire" for a red vodka drink. I knew that I had to go into the office for an hour the next morning; therefore, I brought a bottle of sparkling cider that I sipped on the entire night.

I was dressed as a vampire that night. In my normal life, I tend to do everything by the book, so I always pick naughty, evil, or scary Halloween costumes. It is the one time per year that I can be someone different. Linda gave me a grand tour when I first arrived; I knew some of the people at the party. The guy that I was trying to avoid and I had a brief conversation, but luckily, someone else that I knew walked in and waved at me. We played cool games, like guessing which movie a scene was from. There were dance-offs for the best costumes, and Linda had prizes for every game. She really went all out.

It was getting late, and I needed to leave. Even though I had not used the bathroom yet that night, I had heard from other attendees that, like the rest of the house, it, too, was a scary experience. I placed my cup on a table, headed down the hall to the bathroom, then returned to take my cup to the kitchen, as I did not want to leave Linda's immaculate house dirty. It was clear that she had put a lot of time into preparing for the party. When I returned to the cup, Mike was standing there, dressed as a chef. I had met him briefly earlier that night on the tour of Linda's home. He struck up a conversation about the scary pictures on the counter. A handsome man with a very polite demeanor, he was a refreshing change from the types of men that I had recently met.

Apparently, he and I had met twice the year before at various socials but never connected. However, I could not remember meeting him previously. I asked about his chef costume; it turned out he was a fantastic cook. We had a very long talk about food, and I told him to invite me the next time he had a potluck at his home—I needed to know whether his cooking was as good as he'd told me. He said, "I will need your number to invite you." I walked straight into that one!

The next day, I went to the office for a couple of quick procedures and then went home. I had several errands to do, like laundry and grocery shopping. For a while that day, I thought about Mike, thinking that I would like to see him again. In one of those moments, I heard my phone ring; he had just sent me a text. We texted back and forth for a week. Conveniently, Mike had a potluck at his house the following week, and I was invited. I arrived at his home the following Sunday at 4:45 p.m. Since the dinner didn't start until 5:00 p.m., that gave us some time to talk. He was an immeasurably nice guy; he gave me a tour of his home, as he was almost done grilling. He was right—his lamb chop lollipops were the best that I have ever had. I would later find out that his cooking is as good as a five-star steak house. Wow! I'd found a guy who could cook and who was also attracted to me.

Mike and I went on our first date the following Sunday. He made a brunch reservation at the Café Modern, the restaurant at the Modern Art Museum in Fort Worth. We sat in the restaurant at a table near the glass window. It was beautiful. What I remember most is the look in his eyes when he glanced at me. He still looks at me that way today, even though I am just a person with lots of imperfections. We had a spectacular brunch and then went off to see the impressionists exhibit. Mike was so knowledgeable about the artists, which I admired. When we were done with the museum, he informed me that there was a rose garden not too far away and asked if I wanted to go. I said yes, as I was not on call and was having a good time with him. It turned out that Mike was also very knowledgeable about roses. He had grown them in his yard since childhood and had some in his current backyard. In the rose garden, we took our first photo together on our first date.

At the end of our visit to the rose garden, Mike suggested that we visit the Fort Worth Water Gardens. The architectural design of the gardens is breathtaking. We had such a good time wandering through the various designs. Because it was then time for dinner, we went to Joe T. Garcia's, a popular Mexican restaurant nearby. Although Mike had been there before, I had not. The atmosphere was lively, the service amazing, and the food yummy. Since Mike had spent a lot of time and money on me that day and I did not want to seem ungrateful, I paid for dinner. I got home around 10:00 p.m. that night, having spent about ten hours with a man on a first date, which I had never done before! The greatest part was I could not wait to see him again. Mike texted me good morning every morning and called me every night after our first date. Everything seemed so easy, so natural. I had met my soul mate, and I knew it. Thinking back, the day before the Halloween party had been the second negative pregnancy test, and the day of the Halloween party, I had called my surrogate, Mandy, and the agency and cancelled the remainder of our contract. Perhaps God wanted me to wait to have a child with Mike rather than with donor sperm.

Things went so quickly after our first date. Two weeks later, we were at a Pinot's Palette paint session. Interestingly, we were painting Van Gogh's *Starry Night*. We had seen Van Gogh's self-portrait at the Modern Art Museum on our first date, so it was a nice follow-up in our budding relationship. We were having so much fun that one of the ladies asked us if we were newlyweds; we both looked at each other, smiled, and politely told her we were just dating. Mike and I talked about her comment later that night; our relationship was so natural that strangers had noticed us.

My birthday was that following Monday, but I did not want to tell him that. I did not want him to feel obligated to buy me something since we had been dating for only two weeks at that time. I dropped him off at the airport the Sunday before my birthday because he was heading home to see his dad for Thanksgiving. He gave me a rose from his garden before he left. It was my first flower from him; once it dried, I kept it in an album. A few days later, I left for Thanksgiving to see a friend and his wife in New Jersey. Unable to hold back my excitement, I told them about Mike. I had never told family members or friends about a significant other until I was sure about the relationship. Although I had only been dating Mike for two weeks, however, it felt right.

We both returned from Thanksgiving on Saturday and saw each other that night. I told him that I was in love with him even though it had been only three weeks since our first date. Without hesitation, he said it right back to me. It had taken me six months before I told Ron that I loved him, and that had been after careful thought: we had been dating for six months, and I enjoyed his company, so surely I should be in love with him. But it was different and spontaneous with Mike. I was falling so fast and so hard for a really good man.

Mike and I were on the dating fast track. That Christmas, we bought a tree together, and his dad came into town to visit. I took his dad on a one-on-one date with me to the Perot Museum because I wanted to spend time with the man who had raised Mike. Mike's mom had died of cancer many years before we met; even though neither she nor her dad had ever smoked a day in their lives, they both died of lung cancer. Mike's dad was and still is an extraordinarily pleasant man. I went on their family vacation to Mazatlán, Mexico, in late January. We were sitting in DFW Airport, waiting for our plane at the gate, when a lady noticed Mike and me. She told him that she could see that his girlfriend was really into him. We both smiled when she made that comment; we both knew exactly where things were heading!

Mike proposed to me four months after our first date. Although I knew it was coming, I was not sure when it would happen. He had asked me about my thoughts on marriage when we returned from Mazatlán. His proposal was more over the top than the first date. Mike flies planes for fun and belongs to a flying club here in DFW. One Saturday in early March, we went up for a ride, my first time in a plane with him as the pilot. He had talked about taking me up for a flight; however, we had to wait for a good day when the weather would cooperate and I was not on call. I did not know what to expect. He took me for a spin over my house, giving me a full aerial view—what a surreal experience. Then we changed directions and flew over Love Field into Downtown Dallas and near the city skyline. I got an aerial view of Reunion Tower, where we'd had dinner on Valentine's Day, as well as Bank of America Plaza, Renaissance Tower, Comerica Bank Tower, JPMorgan Chase Tower, Fountain Place, the Sheraton Dallas Hotel, and the Omni Dallas Hotel. It was so amazing. We then hovered the plane facing west to watch the sunset, a magnificent sight to see from a plane. Mike wanted to give me a chance to hold the yoke (the wheel on a plane used for steering). I thought I would hold the yoke in front of me while he was the one really doing the work, but I held and steered the yoke while maneuvering the foot pedals. Even though I was scared and could feel my heart pounding, I was doing a good job. In the corner of my left eye, I saw Mike fumbling for something on his left side, but I could not turn my head to take a good look since I had to keep my eyes to the front of the plane. I could not understand what could be important enough to be fumbling for when he should have been continuing to make sure that I was steering properly. Mike then said, "You are doing a great job. You make a good copilot. Will you be my copilot for life?"

I replied, "Huh?"

He then pulled out an engagement ring. My only response was, "Are you kidding me? You are going to propose now, when I need to concentrate on flying?" Laughing, I quickly took the ring, put it on my finger, and then returned my focus to flying the plane. Mike looked at me oddly, but I understood his look. I said, "Of course, yes, I will marry you." I smiled at him, and he took over flying.

We went back to the airport in McKinney. Once we'd deplaned, he got down on one knee and asked me to marry him again, as he still wanted to propose the old-fashioned way. Flattered, I repeated, "I will marry you today and many million more days to come." He smiled. We returned home and got ready for dinner; Mike had made reservations at Bob's Steak and Chop House in Dallas. As if he had not done enough work already in planning an amazing proposal, we ended the night with a fantastic meal.

Mike tells a funny version of that story. He says that he proposed midair and that if I hadn't said yes, I would have had to exit the plane midair. He is way too funny!

In many ways, Mike makes me wake up every day believing that I live a fairy tale, which is invariably close to the truth. I was lucky to meet a good man—but, like all couples, we are not immune to real-life issues. Mike and I are both human beings capable of mistakes, like all humans. But, somehow, we figured out how to build a relationship based on kindness, trust, and respect. We always strive to treat each other with this kind of reciprocal love. Both Mike and I are the first to admit that marriage requires a lot of patience, dedication, trust, respect, and good communication, and we continue to work at these skills every day. Like many couples, there are days we both think that a happy marital medium only exists in television love stories. Many of my married friends have agreed that marriage is extremely difficult. They were right. Life is incredibly hard. There are some things life throws at you that you survive and that make you stronger, and there are other things that might break you. The strength of the relationship will pull you through the difficult times. It is nice to have someone holding your hand during a crisis. However, stressors can affect a relationship. Mike and I had more stressors coming our way soon, including starting a family.

Nineteen

Before the Marriage

Mike and I had met, dated, and become engaged in just four months. Then there was the excitement of the engagement, with all the calls, texts, emails, and face time with family and friends. A couple of weeks went by, and I realized I needed to tell Mike about my stroke and that I—now we—would need a surrogate. I was hesitant because I was afraid that he would change his mind and not want to get married. However, I have always and continue to believe in honesty, even if honesty meant losing Mike. Two things made my conversation with him easier. One, I already had made the decision to become a parent before I met Mike and had even gone through the process with donor sperm, so I was already comfortable with my own human limitations and had found a way to get around them. Two, we had been only dating for four months. Despite him being the best thing in my life, I could find a way to go back to the way things used to be four months prior. I was at peace with myself and comfortable with all my decisions, but I needed him to make an informed decision. He needed to know everything but also have the option of an out from all this.

We had a long, two-hour phone conversation one night, during which Mike learned about the stroke, the heart defect that had been repaired, and my previous cycles with donor sperm. He knew that I had no physical limitations; he had seen how fast I ran on the treadmill in the gym and how I trumped him in climbing a small mountain in Mazatlán. Although he asked many questions, in the end, he said without hesitation, "Well, if this is what we have to do to have a baby, I am all in." My heart melted. He then added, "I searched my entire life for my unicorn. I am not letting her go. This is just something we have to do together." Mike had a chance to get out of the relationship, but he never considered taking it.

At this point, I was already thirty-eight and a half years old, and Mike was in his midforties, so we needed to act soon, as time was not on our side. Mike went for a semen analysis, which turned out to be not perfect but acceptable for a man his age. We were going to do intracytoplasmic sperm injection (ICSI), in which the sperm would be injected into the egg. ICSI is necessary for male-factor issues, such as poor semen analysis results. His sample was still excellent for ICSI. This time, I intended to do PGT-A screening; I did not want to pay thousands for a gestational carrier if I had only abnormal embryos to put into her uterus. Therefore, I decided we would work on us first. We would need to have good euploid embryos frozen before we found another gestational carrier, so we decided to start banking embryos.

Both of us had furnished homes and did not need anything new. In fact, we needed to get rid of one set of household items. My house was more central in location, and Mike did not like his commute from his home to his workplace. If he lived at my location, he could shave off more than half of his current travel time. We did not want to have a large wedding; planning a stressful wedding was not something that either of us wanted to do, so we planned a very simple ceremony that included a total of seven people, counting the pastor, Mike, and myself. Mike and I were all for basic and easygoing. It was not important to me to have a fabulous dress or a massive wedding. My dress cost $130; it was an elegant bridesmaid dress that I bought in an ivory color and used as my wedding dress. I am an extremely practical, realistic person. I went to three bridal shops one Saturday, and it was my impression that the store representatives were a bit disappointed to have to sell to me, since they must make a commission on sales.

We did our first IVF cycle together—my third round of injections and third retrieval—one month before our wedding ceremony. Mike wanted to learn how to do the injections and insisted that he give them all to me. He wanted to be an active part of this process; I was glad that he was so supportive. Again, I made four to six eggs at the retrieval. Mike's sample that day was poor—much lower than the sample taken just a month before. After the procedures, we had a low quantity of poor-quality embryos. None were euploids. I was disappointed again. We had hit the triple whammy: I was older, with a natural age-related decline in egg quantity and quality; my soon-to-be husband had poor sperm quantity and quality; and we needed a surrogate. What next?

Mike and I had a discussion regarding his samples and decided he should see a urologist. One of the urologists in our area who specialized in male-factor fertility had an office close to Mike's house, so it was easy for Mike to make an appointment. Mike was found to have severe varicoceles—large, dilated veins surrounding the testicles—that needed surgical repair. We all discussed in detail the pros and cons of surgery versus trying another IVF cycle. Even with surgery, we would still need to do IVF with ICSI, but to the doctor's point, performing the varicocelectomies (removal of the varicoceles) would improve Mike's sperm and hence improve our embryo quality. I am still amazed at Mike's courage; he thought about it for just a few seconds before deciding to proceed with the procedure. His surgery was ten days before our wedding ceremony. Talk about bad timing! But we wanted to get the surgery behind us because it could take six to nine months before we saw an improvement in the semen sample and were able to do another IVF-ICSI cycle.

I dropped Mike off for surgery first thing in the morning; I had to work only half of that day and figured his surgery would be done right around lunchtime. Afterward, I walked into the recovery room to find Mike, who was so excited to see me. He looked at me the same way that he'd looked at me on our first date—the same way our son looks at me now. Mike required a lot of ice packs that day but never took any pain medicine the entire time postsurgery. In addition, he only took three days off from work. The following week, he worked from home, never once complaining. I could only imagine how much pain he must have experienced. I insisted on carrying everything since I did not want him to lift anything heavy. Mike decided to cook dinner for me every night despite my instructions to stay off his feet. Mike really wanted children, maybe even more than I did. Now, I wanted a child less for myself and more because it would make my husband immeasurably happy. Mike had spent a lot of time and money on one of his friend's daughters; now he needed his own child to spoil.

Twenty

Conceiving Leo

Mike had frequent follow-up appointments with his urologist and, three months after his surgery, started medications to improve his semen parameters. At six months postsurgery, his semen sample was acceptable for trying another IVF ICSI cycle. I completed another round of injections and a retrieval—my fourth lifetime cycle. Again, I made four to six eggs, and I also thawed my four frozen eggs to create a larger batch. I figured that if I had a larger batch, I would increase the probability of at least one embryo being normal. We had more embryos frozen this time; I was sure that one would be euploid.

The PGT-A results came back: there were no euploids. I was devastated. Up until that point, I'd held it together extremely well around Mike. Every time there was a disappointment, I'd found the courage to move to the next step. When I came home from work that day and told him that there were no euploids, I started to cry hard and loud. I am not sure Mike knew how to react at that time, but I had now done four lifetime retrievals and had no euploids for a transfer. I was done.

By now, I had lost all hope. Hope—the one thing that had gotten me through two massive hurricanes, the deaths of my sisters Nikki and Andromeda, the death of Granny, a stroke, the repair of a heart defect, reconstructive surgery of my right ankle, and the difficulties of pursuing a career in medicine. I had tackled situations that were more life and death and had larger consequences than my infertility. Yet this felt like my biggest struggle. Since I had lost all hope, all I had now was despair. As a physician, I had been aware of the possibility of such a devastating reaction. I could talk to my husband, family, and friends; I could do exercises and all the things that helped me find my happy place. But in the end, the only thing that could fix everything was a healthy child—something that seemed impossible at that time.

A few days later, our embryologist called me. The biopsies had been done in our IVF lab, but the samples had been analyzed by an independent genetics lab. A genetics lab will typically call embryos either euploid or aneuploid, which is a very black-and-white delineation: euploids can be transferred to the uterus, while aneuploids should not be. The independent lab realized that none of my embryos were euploid, but one of the embryos was a mosaic—an embryo that had both euploid and aneuploid cells. The lab called our embryologist, who later called me. This was my first time learning about mosaics. PGT-A analyzes biopsies of the trophectoderm—the part of the embryo that would eventually become the placenta—but there is no biopsy of the actual embryo. In theory, the embryo and placenta should have the same genetic content. However, many embryos have some abnormal cells initially and then autocorrect to normal. Doing the biopsy on a blastocyst—a later-stage embryo—reduces but does not eliminate the possibility of a mosaic. Depending on where the embryologist sampled the trophectoderm, some normal and abnormal cells might be present. The independent lab automatically called an embryo aneuploid even if only one of the cells was aneuploid and the remaining cells were euploid. This was to avoid transfering potentially abnormal embryos to the uterus. In reality, some mosaics are truly euploid.

We thought about whether or not to transfer this mosaic embryo, which would require signing consent forms indicating that we accepted full responsibility of the outcome, especially since the clinic was not recommending transfer. If we had been transferring the embryo to *my* uterus, I would have been OK with a mosaic and accepted all risks. But we were transferring to another woman. Knowing that the embryo was questionable from the very beginning, we were not sure she would be OK with this. Surrogacy was also an unbelievably expensive process. I did not want to make the financial investment knowing that I had not placed an optimal embryo in the uterus.

I could not do another IVF cycle to try to make euploids because I had now done four lifetime cycles. At this point, I told Mike that we needed to try either donor eggs or adoption. His first question was, "What are donor eggs?" I explained that they are eggs retrieved from an anonymous younger woman, usually in her twenties, and that they would be fertilized with his sperm to form the embryos. We would then test the embryos with PGT-A. If we had euploids, we could then proceed with finding a gestational carrier.

Mike's response was entirely selfless: he would rather adopt than have a child that was not genetically related to his wife. He explained, "I want to look into my child's eyes and see my wife. I want see my wife's quirky behavior in my child."

Then it was my turn to be selfless: "If we used a donor egg, we could use *your* sperm, and the child would be related to at least one of us." We were each only considering the other.

We agreed that we would at least explore the donor egg route. Mike is white, a northern boy from North Dakota who grew up in the Midwest. He enjoys a day that's twenty degrees Fahrenheit with at least two feet of snow outside. He has blue eyes and brown hair, and his skin is pale white. On the other hand, I am an Asian blend: fourth-generation Indian, Pakistani, and Chinese. I am often mistaken for Indian, Middle Eastern, or sometimes Hispanic or black. If it is below eighty degrees Fahrenheit, I need a winter coat. I have dark brown eyes and beautiful olive-brown skin. We wanted a baby that was a blend of our characteristics. Nationally, there are many white donors, some black donors, and some Hispanic donors, but very few Asian donors. In many Asian cultures, using an egg donor is not acceptable. Additionally, not many Asian women voluntarily choose to be donors. However, I did not want a white donor; with a white donor egg and a white husband, I would have a white baby. The last thing I wanted was for people to ask me if I were the nanny. Mike also wanted a donor that looked like me, so I decided to look for an Indian or Middle Eastern donor.

After contacting several agencies, I found a total of two donors of Indian origin in Texas. Just like all patients, the donors' identities remained anonymous to me. I showed the two Asian donor profiles to Mike, but he did not like either, observing that they both looked "too Indian." I was stuck. Was he ready to move to adoption?

A few weeks went by. I brought up the topic numerous times during those weeks, asking Mike what he wanted. He said he wanted our child to be biologically related to us. I explained that I was now six months shy of my fortieth birthday and had done four cycles with no euploid embryos to show for it. Realistically, rolling the dice again did not seem fair to me, as the odds were stacked against me. I had already given it more than a fair shot. In addition, I could not mentally or emotionally handle another negative result. While the sperm does provide 50 percent of the embryo's DNA, the egg is more important than the sperm. With a good, young egg, there would be a better chance of having a good euploid embryo. I tried for weeks to convince Mike to do a donor egg cycle, but he did not want to. He finally said to me, "Can you do one more cycle? If this cycle does not work, I want to proceed with adoption."

Mike did not want to do both a donor egg and a gestational carrier. From his viewpoint, the child would have no connection to his wife. I reminded him that in six months, I planned to celebrate my fortieth birthday: "I am too old." He reminded *me* that my mom had delivered six children, her last when she was thirty-eight years old. In other words, my mom would get pregnant if my dad so much as looked at her too long! Mike said that if we did not have to use a gestational carrier, we probably could have conceived on our own after his surgery; I thought about it for a few days and then agreed that I would do one more cycle.

In reality, I was not hopeful about this fifth cycle; I was doing it only to make my husband happy so he could feel comfortable moving on to the next step. I reminded myself numerous times that if it did not work out, we would move on accordingly. The fifth round of injections and retrieval rolled around. Although I continued to do as many as four different injections daily, I never complained. These were the cards that God had dealt me. I could cry and feel sorry for myself, or I could try to be brave and do it again. I chose the latter. It was helpful to know that if it did not work this time, I would no longer have to do another cycle. Again, I made four to six eggs at retrieval, but only one embryo was good enough to do the PGT-A biopsy and freeze. We had to wait several days for the

PGT-A results. Amazingly, I did not even think about it; I expected it to be abnormal.

On Memorial Day of 2016, the embryologist called me with the PGT-A results. I was very casual about the call since I had lost hope at this point. The embryologist reported that our one embryo was a euploid male. I was elated! I ran to Mike, screaming with joy that we finally had a euploid. Male or female did not matter to us; we were happy that we finally had an embryo to work with.

A single euploid embryo after five egg retrievals. For most women, it does not take five cycles to make a single euploid embryo. Many women do so in the first cycle. Mike and I had a lot working against us—I with my advanced maternal age and, hence, lower egg quantity and quality; Mike with his varicoceles and, hence, lower sperm quantity and quality. In combination, the egg and sperm resulted in a lower quantity and quality of embryos. It really becomes a numbers game: the more eggs and sperm—and, hence, embryos—you have to work with, the higher the chances that at least one embryo will be euploid. We were just in a less optimal situation than most couples. Even though I am a strong-willed woman who really understands the process, I broke down numerous times due to disappointment. I'd only done a fifth cycle because we could not find an egg donor who was right for us and because my husband had asked me to give it one last try.

Twenty One

Finding a Gestational Carrier (Surrogate)

I have used the terms gestational carrier and surrogate interchangeably in this book. "Traditional surrogacy" describes a pregnancy in which the woman carrying the pregnancy is also biologically related to the fetus. Today, however, traditional surrogacy is rarely done in the United States, and generally, the term "surrogacy" presently refers to "gestational surrogacy." This is a pregnancy in which the woman carrying the pregnancy does not have any biological relationship to the fetus. Gestational surrogacy is now the type most commonly used in the United States.

Mike and I had only one embryo to work with, which means we had only one shot at this. We needed to find the right gestational carrier, so I contacted the surrogacy agency that I had previously worked with two years before. We started looking at profiles. I was extremely selective with gestational carriers, especially in light of my previous attempted surrogacy cycle and the fact that I only had one embryo to work with this time. Now, I wanted a gestational carrier who had already done a surrogacy cycle successfully because I needed to know that her body (and hence her uterus) would respond well to the hormonal medications. Naturally, I continued to be selective based on the candidate's medical history, her previous obstetrical history, her personal essays, and whether she lived in Texas.

We looked at the profiles of several gestational carriers; only one was perfect and met all our criteria. I was so excited that we'd found a carrier who was perfect for us. Stacy lived four hours away, and she had two children of her own. Earlier in the year, she had successfully delivered a baby that she carried as a surrogate. Stacy had a graduate degree and worked with animals; she was exceptionally levelheaded; and her answers to the questions in her profile were well thought out. Her records indicated that she'd had a good response to the hormonal medications in her previous surrogacy cycle, and she had had an uneventful pregnancy and delivery. I could not believe that we'd found such a perfect carrier. To this point, I had been familiar only with disappointment. Mike and I skyped with her and her husband, and we absolutely loved them. It felt like a match made in heaven!

Mike and I went to North Dakota to visit his family later that month; while we were there, the agency coordinator called me. There had been a massive change in direction at Stacy's job. Both Stacy and her husband worked for the same company, and they were worried that they both might lose their jobs since the company was not doing well. They might have to move. Although Stacy was now sending out her résumé to various other companies, she was still interested in being our surrogate. I felt terrible for Stacy, but her life was too stressful and unpredictable now. Additionally, stress would not be good for the pregnancy. We had found the right carrier, but she was in the wrong place and time of her life to do another surrogacy cycle. She did not know her future or how long the unpredictability would last. Mike and I again skyped with Stacy and her husband; both she and I knew that we could not continue down this path. The good news was that we had not yet signed any legal documents, so it was easy to make a clean break.

Mike and I viewed several more profiles, but none of them were exactly what we were looking for. Ruth's profile did strike me, though. She had had a massive car accident as a child yet still went on to live a normal life and have three children. Ruth and her husband lived only a thirty-minute drive from us. Her profile was perfect, except that she had never done a surrogacy cycle. We met Ruth and her husband for coffee, and we loved them. I was still worried about this being her first surrogacy cycle, though, so I wanted her to have a full medical evaluation before we proceeded with legal documents. She went in for the evaluation; it turned out that her three previous deliveries had been complicated by preterm labor symptoms. On imaging, her uterus was not ideal. She had failed the medical evaluation, and we were devastated.

Onward. We looked at a few more profiles; again, none seemed perfect. There was another woman whose profile seemed excellent, except that this would be her first surrogacy cycle also. She lived in Houston and had family in DFW, so she could visit her family while she was here for testing. We decided to skype with her; she was extraordinarily nice. Based on the first interview, she seemed to be a great person. However, Mike did not feel that she was a good match for us. Not surprisingly, when we heard back from the surrogacy agency, we learned that this gestational carrier did not feel that we were a good match for her either.

All my staff members knew what I was going through. One of them had also done IVF to have her son; she told her sister, who had four children at the time, about me, and her sister reached out to me. She'd had no problems conceiving or carrying her own children, but she had never done a surrogacy cycle. We decided to meet her and her husband for coffee, and again, we really liked them; they were such selfless people. But after the meeting, both the sister and I decided that we were not a good match. We had different views on what would happen to the pregnancy in the rare event that certain circumstances arose. This was very important to Mike and me. We needed someone who was aligned with us on our views. The sister wished me good luck with my search. I am still flattered that my staff member asked her sister to carry my pregnancy—it speaks highly of both her and her sister.

One of my friends is a gay man. He is happily married to his partner, and they used a surrogate to have their twins. In one of our many discussions about surrogacy, he told me that he and his partner had known they needed both a donor egg and a surrogate to have children. This was hard for me to swallow. Of course they needed both a donor egg and a surrogate; they were both men. I am a woman whose eggs were on their last leg, and despite having a viable uterus, it was not safe for me to carry my own pregnancy. It had been an easy decision for him to pursue egg donation and surrogacy, but it was not an easy decision for me. I had many feelings of inadequacy about having my own children. My friend and his partner did one cycle and made many normal embryos. On the other hand, I did five cycles to make one euploid embryo. This friend was kind enough to mention me to his surrogate, but she was not interested in doing another surrogacy cycle at that time. However, she knew a few other women that might be interested. These women were not part of an agency but did this independently. When he called me with their details, I thanked him for such an effort in helping me, but I did not feel that any of them was a good match. I know that I was being too picky; however, I had only one embryo and hence only one shot at this.

Mike and I contacted the surrogacy agency again—back to square one. We found an almost ideal candidate; the only problem was that she lived in Oregon. Mike did not want her to live so far from us that we could not make it to an emergent event in a timely fashion. Another Texas surrogate was forty years old and had five children of her own. As a massage therapist, she was also on her feet a lot, which was a cause of concern for us. Another surrogate, Kayla, had three children of her own. Although she had not done a surrogacy cycle, all three of her children were IVF babies. She knew how the IVF process worked. I would be able to see how her body had responded to the medications by looking at her old records. This candidate lived four and a half hours from us in Texas, and she also had a military background, which said a lot about her discipline and dedication. We liked her on paper. But would we like her in person? We would have to work with her for about a year or longer, and we would have to trust her to carry our most prized possession for nine months!

We skyped with Kayla the day before my fortieth birthday. I had worked a long day that Wednesday, and we had plans to fly out bright and early Thursday morning for a few days to celebrate my fortieth. I enjoyed doing the Skype interviews because it was so much easier to see someone during the conversation without having to drive or fly a long distance. At this point, doing these interviews had become routine for Mike and me, such that, sadly, we had become very good at the process. Although we were ready to just find a gestational carrier, we wanted to be sure that we found the right person.

We had a lot in common with Kayla and her husband, Peter. Kayla was originally from the Midwest but had grown up in Hawaii, where her parents still lived; Peter's family roots were in Puerto Rico, which is an island neighboring St. Croix, the island where I grew up.

Like Mike and I, Kayla enjoyed reggae music. Peter played music; Mike played several instruments in grade school. Furthermore, Kayla was in the military, like I had been, and was, like me, highly dedicated and disciplined. They aligned so well with us in terms of personalities, interests, and, more importantly, views on what to do if something went wrong with the pregnancy.

Kayla knew what it was like to want children and not have them. She had been in her early thirties when they did IVF, and she had made many nice embryos. They'd transferred two embryos on the first transfer and had a healthy twin delivery several months later. I was impressed with her obstetrician, who'd delivered her twins by vaginal delivery. The twin delivery was her first pregnancy; first pregnancies tend to be more difficult than subsequent ones. It said a lot about her body that she had been able to carry and deliver twins at term by vaginal delivery. It also said a lot about her doctor's skill as a competent physician. Kayla did an FET cycle with her next pregnancy; one embryo was transferred, and she delivered a healthy baby a few months later. With our surrogacy cycle, she would essentially do another FET cycle, like in her previous pregnancy. She would use the same medications to prepare her body before the embryo was thawed and transferred.

I asked Kayla why she wanted to be a gestational carrier. She responded, "I, too, could not have children the old-fashioned way and needed IVF. Now I experience the joys of being a mother, and I want other women to experience this too." She had made five good embryos, but though she'd had three children, she did not want five. She wanted to be a surrogate twice, giving birth to two babies to make up for not using her two remaining embryos. I asked questions about her military obligations. She was now a stay-at-home mom and only did military training once per month. In all her previous pregnancies, her monthly training sessions had been nonstrenuous.

Everything happened so quickly after our first interview. In less than a month, Kayla came to DFW for her medical evaluation. She had a hysteroscopy to evaluate her uterus and passed her medical exam. We met her for lunch, our first time meeting Kayla in person. She was a tall, beautiful woman with a great sense of humor. Mike and I loved her.

Medical clearance and psychological clearance are often completed before one starts the legal documents for surrogacy. Kayla passed the medical exam, which indicated that she was a viable candidate to be a gestational carrier. Psychological clearance was necessary to be sure all parties were comfortable with the process. Naturally, both Mike and I were comfortable having another person involved in our childbearing. My stroke had been at age twenty-three; at that age, I had been devastated that I might not have children. I was now forty years old; I had had enough time to think about this decision. However, I'd done more than just decide to use a surrogate. I had found peace with the fact that I had to trust someone else to take care of my child for nine months. Many of my friends asked whether I was jealous that I would not have that bond with my child. I was not jealous of Kayla, even though I did mourn the fact that I would never be able to feel my own child kicking inside of me. But this was my reality. If there was one thing my upbringing had taught me, it was that I always needed to be realistic about my situation. Things could always be worse. That was another of the many traits that I liked about Kayla: she was also amazingly realistic. She already had three children, and she did not want to raise any more. There was no doubt in my mind about her relinquishing the child after birth.

Once we had both medical and psychological clearance, it was time to work on the legal paperwork. Everything went very smoothly; the documents delineated all aspects of the pregnancy in detail. In addition to the gestational documents, our attorney would need to file a prebirth order a few months before delivery. In the past, prebirth orders did not exist. Generally, if a woman delivered a baby, the birth certificate would be in her name. Couples would then have to turn around and adopt their own child, even if the child were biologically related to them. With a prebirth order, we would have an order from a judge that we could take to the hospital at delivery and that would prove that we were the parents of the baby. The original birth certificate could then be printed in our names.

Many people have asked me what choosing a surrogate is like. I often tell them it is like finding your significant other while also doing a job interview. You want someone who is aligned with you on so many levels; you have to be able to work with this person; and you and this woman will have a very intimate relationship. But, at the same time, you do not want someone who has such a relaxed personality that she does not pay attention to details, as you are trusting essentially a stranger with a precious possession. I had achieved many things in life, but my greatest achievement was my tiny, microscopic embryo, which I hoped would someday be a living, breathing infant that I would hold in my arms. Yes, I spent a lot of time being extraordinarily selective of the gestational carrier, but once I selected someone that I felt would treat my child the way that I would, I stopped worrying. We had already vetted her healthy lifestyle and were aligned with her on all decisions concerning pregnancy. Therefore, because I already had a good sense of her personality, I never micromanaged her day-to-day activities. For example, I never told her what to eat, wear, or do, and I only spoke to her during her doctor's appointments or if something came up. Otherwise, I allowed her to live her life, and she never burdened me with anything or made me feel guilty in any way.

Kayla thanked me for this numerous times throughout the pregnancy. She'd joined a surrogacy support group, and a few surrogates had told her that their experiences had not been as good as hers. We had a mutually respectful relationship.

Twenty Two

The Pregnancy: Why Does It Feel Like There Is Nothing Easy in My Life?

Now that all the legal documents had been signed, Kayla started the gestational carrier cycle. She took medications to prepare her uterus, and her body had a positive response. Fortunately, she never once complained about taking the medications; they were the same ones she had used for her pregnancies. Kayla was able to do ultrasound and blood-work monitoring near her home, which was exceptionally helpful for her since she was the primary caregiver of her three young children.

Once her uterus was ready, Kayla came into DFW for the transfer, which was scheduled for midday. Embryos are typically thawed first thing in the morning, observed for growth in culture for a few hours, and then transferred. Both Mike and I worked half days that day. I could not sleep the night before because I was excited and nervous at the same time—excited because I was one step closer to having a child, nervous because I knew everything that could go wrong. The embryo would have to thaw and survive the thaw; the transfer would need to be a seamless procedure; and the embryo would then have to find a cozy spot in the uterus to implant and grow. Then there were numerous things that could go wrong during the nine months of incubation and delivery. However, I was unbelievably realistic and calm throughout the process. With every step, both Mike and I were grateful to move on, but we did not want to celebrate anything until we could hold a living, breathing child in our arms. We had had too many disappointments throughout this process, and we did not want to get our hopes up.

That day, we met Kayla in the holding room before the embryo transfer. We were so excited to see her that we took several photos to document this stage. The embryologist gave us a photo of our embryo. It was time. Kayla had done transfers before with her previous pregnancies. Embryo transfers are amazingly easy procedures, much like a Pap smear. The only uncomfortable part is the need to have a full bladder. Luckily, the transfer was routine for her; what was not routine was that this was not genetically her embryo. One of my initial requirements in searching for a gestational carrier had been someone who had done surrogacy before. While Kayla had not done a surrogacy cycle before, she had done a fresh IVF cycle and an FET cycle. This was an FET cycle similar to what had been done with her previous pregnancy, so Kayla did extraordinarily well during the transfer. We saw on the ultrasound monitor the flash when the embryo was injected—a small flash on the screen as the bubble of air and medium in which the embryo was suspended was injected into the uterus. Finally, it was all done! Only time would tell if the embryo implanted.

A nurse and one of my dear friends led a meditation for Kayla at her request. Many women do acupuncture, meditation, or some other form of relaxation after a transfer. My friend now did post-transfer meditations after a glorious career as an infertility nurse. She believed that, many times, our mental state can influence our body; she is a proponent of the mind-body connection in dealing with fertility. She and I had worked together before she retired from being a fertility nurse. Since her retirement, she and I have attained an amazing friendship, and I am lucky to have her in my life. Several years ago, I wrote a chapter titled "Does Psychiatric Diagnosis Affect Fertility Outcomes?" for the book *Women's Reproductive Mental Health Across the Lifespan*, published in 2014. Since I valued her opinion on mental health and fertility, my dear friend helped by previewing one of the earlier versions of this chapter. Her review brought us closer. When Mike and I got engaged, I told her that Mike and I were not interested in having a large ceremony, so she recommended her friend, a pastor, who married Mike and me. Since the church that I attended was too large and did not have the right kind of setup, we were married in a small chapel inside the church that our friend attended every Sunday. Coincidentally, my home in DFW was in her old neighborhood. I had invited her and her husband over for dinner one night, and they told me that their old house was just down the road. This is truly a small world. She was another angel that God sent to me, and I am lucky to have her in my life. When my friend told me that she really liked Kayla, it confirmed that Kayla and I were a perfect match.

Kayla stayed in DFW for one night after the embryo transfer because we wanted her to get as much rest as possible. Driving almost five hours to DFW, doing the transfer, and driving another five hours back would have been too stressful. Kayla's husband, Peter, did her progesterone injections, which are necessary to sustain a pregnancy. The progesterone injections are intramuscular injections given in the gluteus muscle. It is difficult to self-administer progesterone injections because of the angle required to reach your back; also, it is a large needle that goes into the muscle. Peter did not come with Kayla to the embryo transfer; he stayed at home to take care of their three children. Kayla needed someone to give her the progesterone shot before she left to go home the day following the transfer, so I stopped by her hotel room to give her the injection. It was so easy for her—she did not fuss about the shot at all—and by giving one shot, I felt like I was some part of the process. After her progesterone injection, Kayla checked out of the hotel and drove home. Before she left, she did mention that she had finally gotten one good night of sleep without having to deal with three screaming kids!

We had to wait ten days after the transfer before the first pregnancy test—probably the longest ten days of my life. I had optimized every aspect of this pregnancy that I had control over. We'd done PGT-A genetic testing of the embryos before selecting the right embryo for transfer, and I'd chosen the most ideal gestational carrier possible. The transfer had gone smoothly; however, even with everything optimized, there was still only about a 60–80 percent chance of a positive pregnancy test. I knew too well that there was no 100 percent guarantee of this working. I was once again reminded what it was like to be in my own patients' shoes. There were still so many things we could not control. Above all, I was not optimistic; I was realistic. I'd already had two failed pregnancy tests with the first surrogate three years earlier, so I never allowed myself to get my hopes up for fear of another disappointment.

Kayla completed the pregnancy blood test at a local laboratory near her home, and the results were then faxed to DFW. My entire staff knew that it was my destiny day. No one wanted to say anything to me, as they were just as nervous as I was. However, many of them were unbelievably hopeful. Hope was something that had seemed to slowly slip away from my hands. It is terrible what repetitive disappointment can do to someone. My front-desk staff received the fax and brought it to my office, with the results facing down, while I was seeing a patient in another room. When I returned to my desk, I found the paper facedown. I knew what was on the other side, but I was hesitant to turn the sheet to face upward. Nervously, I took one big breath and turned the paper over.

The pregnancy test was positive!

It was not *just* positive; the pregnancy hormone measured, beta human chorionic gonadotropin (BHCG), was a high value. I felt myself exhale. In the excitement, I did not have time to call Mike to give him the news. All my staff ran to my office to tell me congratulations. They all had seen the results when the fax came through. My office phone then rang. One of the nurses at another location had called after checking the lab website about a dozen times that morning, hoping that she would see the results; she had been on the lookout for them because she knew that, three years prior, I had had two negative results. When she saw the results—at right around the same time that the fax came over—she was excited for Mike and me. I called Mike about thirty minutes later. He was excited at the good news and rightly joked that he was probably the thirtieth person to find out.

As per standard protocol, Kayla had several repeated pregnancy-hormone blood tests, and her numbers continued to increase appropriately. Once the hormone values were high enough, we scheduled a pregnancy ultrasound. We decided to have her sonogram done at a local facility near her home. Kayla lived almost five hours from us, and she had already been to DFW three times during this process. She had three young children at home. Kayla was their primary caregiver since her husband worked during the week. They did not have any family in Texas, so every time she came to DFW, she had to find a babysitter for the entire day. Although we paid for her babysitter, the drive and the thought of leaving her kids with a stranger for such a long time were difficult for her. So, we suggested that she have the sonogram at a facility near her home, even though this caused some of my staff to be upset with me because they wanted to be there for it. I cannot begin to describe how incredibly lucky I was to have my staff.

Mike and I drove to Austin for Kayla's sonogram. She was almost eight weeks pregnant and already had a tiny baby bump. Just as at all her previous visits, Mike insisted that he stand at the head of the examining table—he wanted to see only the ultrasound screen, not Kayla's private parts. On the sonogram, we saw our tiny baby, less than one inch in length at that time. Interestingly, Kayla was just as anxious that day as we were. She was already very emotionally invested in our child. I was again reminded that I had picked the right person to carry our child. We all were at ease once we heard the baby's heartbeat.

At around ten weeks of pregnancy, Kayla initiated prenatal care with her obstetrician. This was my first time meeting him, but I had heard so many good things about him. Mike came with me to the first prenatal visit. I absolutely loved her physician; he is such a per-fect blend of talented and skillful yet very personable and likeable.

His office was in one of the professional buildings adjacent to the hospital, which worked out well for him since he could see patients and be close to the hospital for deliveries. We also liked that we had established a driving pattern to the location. Over the next several months, we would continue to familiarize ourselves with the area. At Kayla's first prenatal appointment, the doctor did a sonogram that confirmed that the pregnancy was continuing to grow appropriately. Everything seemed to be going just right. I hoped that we were now in the clear from disappointments.

Unfortunately, we were not in the clear. A few weeks later, Kayla had heavy bleeding. Naturally, she called me. While I usually tried to be just the intended mother in my relationship with her, I now had to put on my doctor's hat. I reassured her that, many times, women have bleeding in the first trimester and continue to have normal pregnancies with good deliveries. Bleeding in the first trimester is quite a common complaint and is usually self-resolving. I told her to stay off her feet, to do no heavy lifting, and to minimize her activities. She was fine for a few hours, but then the bleeding worsened. This time, she decided not to call me but to go to the emergency room. A few hours later, she called to say she could not take it any longer; she was worried that she was having a miscarriage. An ultrasound in the ER showed that the baby was still there and still had a heartbeat. She also now had a subchorionic hematoma. A subchorionic hematoma is a collection of blood near the pregnancy. She called her doctor's office and made a follow-up appointment.

I attended that appointment. Her subchorionic hematoma was seven centimeters; while I had seen subchorionic hematomas before, I had never seen one that large—larger than the pregnancy. The doctor told me that if he had not already known that we transferred just one embryo, he would have mistaken the subchorionic hematoma for a larger second sac. There was no second baby, though, and we had already had several normal sonograms just weeks before. My doctor brain started to work overtime; I knew what Kayla's obstetrician was going to say. He told us that a subchorionic hematoma this large could lead to loss of pregnancy early on or, later, to preterm labor and delivery. He then asked Mike and me to leave the room, after which he told Kayla to avoid all strenuous activity, including having intercourse.

I felt so guilty. This woman was not only carrying my child but now could not have sex with her husband and had to avoid lifting her children. What was I putting her through? And we had many more months to go until delivery. She'd had two uncomplicated pregnancies, including one with twins; this was certainly more than she'd thought she was signing up for. There was nothing I could do to fix this. I felt helpless.

Kayla's doctor then asked Kayla to have weekly appointments, as he wanted to evaluate her bleeding and see whether the subchorionic hematoma would resolve. I went to all the visits because I needed to see the sonograms for myself. Kayla had another large episode of bleeding the following week, but she did not go to the ER that day since she had an appointment with her obstetrician in a few days. The sonogram showed a healthy, growing pregnancy despite the large subchorionic hematoma.

Kayla continued to have sporadic bleeding for the next several weeks. Three weeks following the initial bleeding episode, her sonogram showed that the subchorionic hematoma was resolving. It no longer looked like fresh blood; it was, however, still at seven centimeters and continued to be larger than the baby. I felt better about the new findings but continued to be cautiously optimistic. The weekly visits and the thought of losing the pregnancy were equally as disturbing to Kayla as they were to me. She felt personally responsible for my child even though I'd reminded her numerous times that these things could happen. Once the bleeding had completely subsided, we sent her a gift card for a spa day. She was so happy to have a day to herself with no worries about bleeding or screaming children.

Mike was also having problems coping with the recent events. One night, he and I were at home, and Mike was watching an episode of *Jimmy Kimmel Live!* in which Kimmel gave detailed information about his son needing surgery for a congenital heart defect. While Kimmel could afford to pay for his son's medical care, he used his story and platform to discuss his frustrations with politics and their negative impact on health care, which could leave less fortunate children unable to get appropriate medical care. Mike started to talk about this episode as he watched it; he was devastated. My dear husband started to sob about all the uncertainties of our current pregnancy. Like Kimmel, we were also having a son. My own heart defect was the reason we were in this predicament in the first place. Mike was now worried that our son, too, would have a heart defect and potentially have complications. I consoled Mike several times by reminding him that my heart defect had not been genetic and had since been fixed. Kimmel's son's heart defect had nothing to do mine or with our pregnancy. After a very long night of Mike staring at the television and repeatedly going over what I had just told him, he was finally able to go to sleep.

This pregnancy was already affecting us; disappointments were our new normal. It seemed that Mike was getting himself mentally ready for all forms of disappointment. He took things different-ly than I did. Because I am in the medical field and had a fairly good grasp of our problems, I had to be the strong one, but Mike's reactions were always a good reminder of what my own patients go through. They do not always understand everything, and even when they understand the situation, many do not have a support system to help them pull through it. Many are too afraid to tell their family and friends that they are going through fertility treatments, so when things do not go right for them, they have no one to lean on. Mike and I had each other to lean on, but we did not have family or friends that we could lean on at that time. We had not yet told anyone about the baby due to the uncertainty of whether it would come to fruition.

Apart from my office staff, no one knew that we were expecting. My parents knew about my stroke, about the heart defect that I'd had repaired, and about my need for a gestational carrier. They were also aware that I had been freezing embryos for several cycles, that I had one good embryo, and that I'd been looking for a gestational carrier. I had not told them that I had found the carrier and that she was pregnant. Because I was so tired of disappointment and of having to explain everything to everyone repeatedly, I now avoided the topic. My mom, however, suspected. She knew my level of self-motivation and strength. Although she had inquired several times, I had avoided the conversation. In fact, I avoided it so well that she suspected I was afraid to tell her.

Kayla was about sixteen weeks pregnant by the time I told my family. They were very happy for me but knew the road was going to be a long one. My two nephews, four and five years old at that time, heard my parents talking, so they were excited. The older nephew—my brother's son—understood that he would soon have another cousin. He had three half brothers; however, he did not know I was not pregnant. He saw me once per year, at best, when

I visited St. Croix, and he did not understand the concept of a gestational carrier. The younger nephew—my sister's only child—did not understand the idea of a cousin; he thought that he would soon have a brother. Both nephews were excited about a baby, though, which was a term they understood well. After my first conversation with my family regarding the gestational carrier, they began wanting an update every time I spoke to them. On every phone call, my nephews asked when the baby would come. The older nephew knew the months of the year and understood that he had to wait until November, so every time I called, he would say the months of the year in chronological order until he got to November. The younger nephew did not understand months, but on every phone call, he asked when he would be able to play with the baby.

Mike's family, on the other hand, did not know much at all. They knew that Mike had had surgery two years prior and understood why he'd had the surgery. Therefore, they were aware that we were actively working on the baby-making process. They also knew that Mike had married a fertility doctor and that, therefore, I might be orchestrating our fertility plans. Mike's dad was heading over to visit us for Father's Day; Mike wanted to tell him in person when he arrived in Texas. Once his dad had learned about the pregnancy, Mike then planned to tell his other family members.

Mike's dad showed up to our home the Friday before Father's Day. He had driven alone all the way from Illinois, a trip he had completed numerous times in the past. But something was different this time. Mike came home early that day to meet his dad, and I came home later. When I first saw my father-in-law, John, that night, I suspected something was wrong even though I had not seen him in over a year. In the last year, Mike had heard that his dad had had several falls; he had recovered from them, however, and did not want Mike to worry. Still, he showed up to our home with fresh bruises on his right arm, right hand, and the right side of his chest, having fallen the night before at a gas station in Wichita Falls, Texas. He complained that he was getting more and more clumsy with each day. Although he had initially increased volunteering at his church in Illinois after his wife died of cancer, as a way for him to get his mind off of her while still socializing, in the last year, he had scaled back these activities. He had also lost a significant amount of weight, was frail, had gait issues following a hip replacement, and was fighting diabetes. We wondered what was causing his frequent dizziness and falls.

That night during dinner, we told John that we were expecting a child, sharing all sorts of details so that he could understand every-thing. He was so excited. He did not have any grandchildren, and he wanted some. Father's Day was extra special that year for John; he was now celebrating that he was going to be a grandfather. Mike and I, however, refused to personally celebrate Father's or Mother's Day because we did not want to jinx anything.

We told John that we were heading to Austin the following week for Kayla's second-trimester anatomy scan. This was an ultrasound typically done around twenty weeks of gestation. Although John had planned to visit us for only one week, he decided to stay a second week to see the sonogram, which was scheduled at 8:00 a.m. on a Friday morning. Mike and I worked full days on Thursday, figuring that we would drive Thursday night and stay at a local hotel overnight. We could then go to the sonogram first thing in the morning and drive home later that day. On Thursday, both Mike and I came home from work, quickly ate an early dinner with his dad, and decided to leave once the evening traffic had subsided.

We left just after 6:00 p.m. Since Thursdays were my long procedure days, I was exhausted; luckily, Mike was driving this time, his dad riding in the front passenger seat while I sat in the back, hoping to take a short nap. However, I had drunk a diet Coke, and it had done its job: I was not only alert but needed to go to the bathroom—caffeine is an effective diuretic. Initially, the urge to go was not bad, so I decided that I could wait until we had driven about two hours, which would break up the drive with a rest stop.

In Waco, we stopped at a McDonald's. By this time, I really needed to empty my bladder. As soon as Mike parked the car, I ran into McDonald's, straight to the bathroom, leaving Mike and his dad in the car. I'd made it into a stall when I heard the bathroom door bang open and Mike say, in a serious, emergent voice,

"Dorette, I need you to come quickly." I knew something bad had happened.

John was lying on his back in the parking lot, Mike and several other people surrounding him. I asked someone to call an ambulance and ran over to assess his condition. He was breathing and had a pulse; however, he was not responding. After I called out to him numerous times while applying a sternal rub, he finally opened his eyes and started talking. I surmised that if his blood sugars were low, that might have caused his fall, so I ran back into McDonald's and got a cup of orange juice for him to drink to bring the sugars back up.

By the time the ambulance arrived, John seemed to be responsive. It turned out that he had been walking into McDonald's when another person cut him off and walked in front of him, causing him to lose his balance and fall directly backward, hitting the back portion of his head. We were perplexed about why he had lost his balance. The emergency medical technicians (EMTs) checked his sugar level, which was normal. They then took him to Baylor Scott & White Medical Center–Hillcrest in Waco, which was just a seven-minute drive away. Coincidentally, this was the hospital that my first gestational carrier had intended to deliver at if she had conceived. It is amazing how life comes full circle.

The doctor told us that a CT scan had been normal. He cleaned the wound on the back of John's skull and put three staples in his head. When the doctor realized that I was also a physician, he handed me a staple remover and told me that I could remove the staples in about a week if the wound had closed.

We left the hospital at 11:00 p.m., about three hours since we had pulled into the McDonald's parking lot. Even though we were all tired, we still had two more hours of driving to do. Mike and I kept each other awake, our exhaustion from both having worked a full day now compounded by his dad's accident. We pulled into the hotel's parking lot around 1:00 a.m. By the time we'd checked in, brushed our teeth, and made sure John was tucked in for the night, it was almost 2:00 a.m. Even so, we needed to be up around 6:00 a.m. for all three of us to shower, eat breakfast, and make it to Kayla's 8:00 a.m. appointment in a timely fashion.

My alarm chimed at 6:00 a.m.; a few hours of sleep had not been enough. I am a health enthusiast. I exercise, eat right, and do not take any substances of any sort. Although I usually do not drink coffee in the morning, I decided this was going to be a morning for coffee. After breakfast, we headed over to the clinic. This was the first time I'd really looked at John's head in daylight; he had clotted blood all over his beautiful white hair and looked like he had been in a fight the night before. It was our first time at this clinic; we were seeing a maternal-fetal medicine (MFM) specialist for the anatomy scan. Because it was a large medical center with many buildings, it was not clear which building we should go into, so Mike dropped me off. I called Kayla to locate her, found her, and notified Mike and his dad. A few days earlier, I had told Kayla that my father-in-law was visiting, and she'd had no problem with John attending the ultrasound. Now, I told Kayla all about the accident the night before. When John met Kayla, he, too, immediately liked her. An exceptionally grateful man, he thanked her immensely for carrying his grandson.

When they called us back, Kayla and her party of three proceeded to the sonogram room, where we informed the nurse who the rest of us were in relation to Kayla. The facility was either a new facility or a recently remodeled one, and the sonogram was an updated model that also had the ability to do four-dimensional images. We asked for pictures, so the kind sonographer told us that she would give us a CD of the images at the end of the exam. She then proceeded with the sonogram. I cannot explain what it was like to see my son during this ultrasound; I could not take my eyes off the screen. He was a real person growing inside Kayla. John was so happy to see his grandson, and he repeatedly expressed his thanks to Kayla. Mike had his phone out, taking still images and videos. It was an amazing moment for all of us. We forgot how tired we were and what a long night we'd had the night before.

The subchorionic hematoma was still there, and still seven centimeters, but clotted. Kayla needed a vaginal sonogram to look at her cervical length and assess the subchorionic hematoma in more detail. She said that it was fine for me to stay but that the men needed to leave. After everyone left, I offered to wait outside until she was undressed and draped with the clinical sheet. Outside the room, I walked over to Mike and John; Mike's eyes were bloodshot. I asked if he was OK. He claimed that he was fine, but it was clear that his eyes were bloodshot from crying, not lack of sleep. My husband had many tears of joy because he was going to be a dad. After that day, Mike began speaking so much about the bonding activities that he and his son would be able to do. For him, it was now real.

I returned to the room. Fortunately, Kayla's cervix was long, with no indication of preterm dilation, and the subchorionic hematoma was stable. There was a marginal placental cord insertion, but that was not something to worry about since the baby was growing appropriately. Normally, the placental cord inserts in or near the central portion of the placenta. A marginal placental cord insertion means the cord has inserted within two centimeters of the placental disc's edge. The biggest concern with marginal placental cord insertion is that there can be diminished blood supply to the baby, potentially causing impaired growth and development. The MFM physician gave Kayla the same precautions her obstetrician had given her several weeks earlier and recommended that we return for a repeat scan in eight weeks to check on the baby's growth.

We wished Kayla a good day and started our drive back to DFW. On the way home, I sat in the back seat, looking up and calling all the cord blood banks that I could find. I needed to do my research, as I wanted to bank both cord blood and tissue. Granny had always told me that time is important, so I made good use of my time researching during the drive. I assessed the efficacy and cost of each bank, and by the time we got home, I had decided which we should use.

On our drive back to DFW, we stopped at the Harley-Davidson, which provided a nice break to stretch our legs. Mike also wanted to get a new pair of shades since he had lost his nice Harley-Davidson shades a few weeks earlier. I rode on the back of Mike's Harley once when we were dating, but I prefer that he drive his car because I am extremely risk averse. When we got married, I promised Mike that I would not take away his Harley or his love of flying planes. However, once we had children, I wanted him to cut back on the risky hobbies without stopping them. We agreed that he could ride his Harley to work on the back roads but not on the freeway, where cars moved at excessive speeds. He has thanked me numerous times for not making him give up two things that he really enjoys. While we were at the Harley store looking for Mike's new shades, one of the store clerks approached me. She had noticed the bloodstain on the back of John's skull, so I had to go through all the details of the previous night's events.

John stayed another extra week so we could observe him. It also allowed me to take out his staples before he returned to Illinois.

His wound had healed well by then, so I removed the staples. The next morning, Mike and I discovered that John had packed all of his luggage into his car and was getting ready to drive back to Illinois. Even though he had intended to stay only one week when he came down, he had now been with us for three weeks. He wanted to go home. Since he was doing much better—even better than when he'd first come down to see us—he started his journey back home to Illinois without our objections. John would later get sick several times in the upcoming months, requiring Mike to make multiple trips and numerous phone calls with caregivers in Illinois. All of this happened while Kayla was pregnant, which added to our anxiety.

One of my best friends was aware of the multiple life events I was juggling at the time and insisted that I write a blog. But I was too afraid; I did not want a sensational story. I wanted a normal, boring life in which everything was easy. This friend also insisted that I have a baby shower, but Mike and I did not want to buy any gifts for the baby—we were afraid that if we bought anything, there would be no baby. After she mentioned the shower so many times, though, I finally gave in and agreed to have one if it was in the last month of pregnancy. This close friend was, in many ways, like another sister to me—one of those angels that God sent my way. She had thrown my engagement party two years earlier. Her sweet smile and enthusiastic positivity were infectious.

Mike and I went to Buy Buy Baby to create a registry. We approached the counter and met a nice woman who was approximately in her early sixties. After we explained to her that we wanted to create a registry, she helped us with the paperwork. She inquired whether we were having a boy or girl and about our due date, of which we were only two and half months shy. When I told her the date, she looked at me strangely, but she was too polite to say anything. Still, I knew what she was thinking. I am a small Asian woman of just over one hundred pounds, and I certainly did not look like I was more than six months pregnant. It was end of summer in DFW, so I was wearing a tank top and shorts; it was not like I was hiding a belly under a winter coat. We shared that we were first-time parents and clueless, so we wanted her to explain everything to us in detail. She spent two hours with us, first creating the registry online and then walking around the store with the registry gun to scan our selected items. There was a huge selection of different brands, and we needed to know which brands to buy.

When we got to the baby bottles and nipples, she went into a discussion of how some bottle nipples mimic a woman's anatomical nipple. Breastfed babies could not tell the difference, so it made switching between breast and bottle easier. She asked me whether I was planning to breast or bottle feed, a question I had not seen coming. Mike quickly interjected, "We plan to exclusively bottle feed." Again, the sweet older woman smiled and was too polite to ask me any details. Perhaps she assumed we were adopting.

Next, we arrived at the diaper-pail aisle. I had not known there were so many diaper pails of different colors, sizes, and mechanisms. The clerk reviewed them with us and then asked us to add one to the registry. Mike and I looked at each other. Since we had no idea what color the room would be and whether it would match, we just selected one randomly. The same thing happened when we visited the stroller aisle; there were too many options, and we had no idea which one we wanted. We chose a stroller randomly based on how we felt steering it. More than two hours went by, but we were far from finishing. There was still another major decision: the crib and bedding. We decided to take a break and planned to return in a few weeks because it was all too overwhelming. Now we knew what first-time parents must go through! It was difficult enough trying to have a baby; now, with the baby almost here, we had to get ready. While I am a physician and took care of my younger brother, this was still all too much. That day at the store, I realized that I was now learning the language of parenthood.

My baby shower was fantastic. It was at the same restaurant where we had held my engagement party. I was amazed at all the fabulous gifts; many of my friends have children and knew exactly what they wanted to buy for me. Numerous items were not even on the registry. I am so grateful to them for their love and support. In addition, since my staff knew about the baby, they threw me two separate baby showers at the two different offices. I was overwhelmed with their kindness. I did most of my surgeries at one of the surgery centers in Dallas; the center staff knew that I was doing a surrogacy cycle, and they also surprised me with a baby shower, which completely caught me off guard. Mike's co-workers planned a baby shower for him, too, so we had a total of five showers. Additionally, several of my patients had learned that I was expecting a baby through IVF and surrogacy, so I received many beautiful gifts from these patients, some of whom had not yet conceived. I asked those patients why they'd brought me gifts when I still needed to give them a baby, and they told me that my kindness and sincerity was all they needed. I realized again that even when everything seemed so difficult in my life, there were many people who cared about me. I was lucky to have kind people in my life.

For a couple of months, it seemed that Mike and I were having smooth sailing with regard to the pregnancy, which gave us enough time to work on his dad's medical concerns. Eight weeks following the anatomy scan, Kayla had a repeat sonogram with the MFM doctor that showed that the baby was continuing to grow well. For the remainder of the pregnancy, she would now see only her obstetrician, who repeated the ultrasound a month following her last MFM ultrasound. This sonogram suggested that the baby had fallen off the growth curve: he had been measuring at 68–70 percent growth on all previous scans, but now he was measuring at 32 percent. The subchorionic hematoma was gone, but there was still the marginal placental cord insertion, which could have been responsible for the drop in growth. The baby looked healthy otherwise. There was no need to rush to delivery, but the pregnancy did need close monitoring. If the monitoring visits were good, there would be a repeat ultrasound in three to four weeks to assess growth. We were now back to uncertainty.

During this time frame, Kayla had weekly biophysical profiles (BPPs) and a fetal nonstress test (NST), which both assessed whether the pregnancy was progressing well. Both were normal. Her doctor did a repeat sonogram four weeks after the previous one; based on this sonogram, the baby had continued to stay around the 32 percent growth rate. I was relieved that the baby's growth was stable; that the pregnancy was still stable on the growth curve with the same doctor and the same machine four weeks later was good news. I stopped worrying. All the worrying was not good for my body; on top of that, I had a severe upper respiratory infection (URI) around this time. Since I did not want Kayla to get sick, I did not go to Kyle, Texas, for this visit. Mike had gone to Illinois to work on some of his father's problems; it was difficult for me because I was always the person taking care of everyone else, but now I was too sick to help anyone. We had only three more weeks until the induction, with Kayla continuing to see her obstetrician weekly. If her weekly visits continued to be normal, we would be on track with the original plan to induce at thirty-nine weeks of gestation.

Twenty Three

Control of Mind over Body

It is amazing how the mind and body are so connected. Because I was so worried about everything happening to Kayla and my father-in-law, my ability to fight off a common URI was diminished. I have always believed in the power of positive thinking and how such a mental state can create a positive life environment. Now, I was doing the opposite—a worn-down mental state was having a negative effect on my body. The upper respiratory infection proved short lived as soon as I decided to rest and take care of myself. All of this was happening just before Halloween, one of my favorite times of the year. Mike and I had met at a Halloween party several years earlier; since then, we'd always celebrated the day. This year, my costume was Wonder Woman. The movie had been a big hit that summer. I ordered my costume online; when it arrived in the mail, I was like a kid who'd just woken up on Christmas Day. I had to try it on and take numerous selfies, which I showed my nurse Yvonne the next day. She knew about all the things I was going through at that time, and she said to me, "You are going dressed as yourself." It was odd how well she knew me; Mike had said the same thing to me when the costume arrived the night before. The excitement of attending my friend's Halloween party wearing the costume placed me in a good mental state. My URI was resolving, and with regard to the pregnancy, I started to see the light at the end of the tunnel. There was a real chance that, in three weeks, I would be a mother!

I spoke to Kayla once per week now that she was going in for weekly visits. She never called me to complain about anything, and in return, I never called to impose on her life. About a week and half before the scheduled induction, she called to tell me that the baby was lower in her pelvis, although she had no symptoms of labor. She did not feel that she needed to go to the hospital. Besides, she lived maybe five or ten minutes from the hospital, so if there were an emergency, she could get there quickly. Mike was worried that Kayla would deliver unexpectedly and that we would miss our son's birth, so he packed a suitcase and left it in his car. He insisted that I pack a suitcase, too, and leave it in my car.

Mike spoke about the baby at least a dozen times per day. He was getting nervous, and his anxiety was infectious; now I was anxious too. But I expressed my anxiety differently. I started having chest pain that was not relieved by any medication or relaxation; I suspected it was related to stress. However, I had also had a stroke at age twenty-three, with a heart defect subsequently repaired. Deciding that I needed to get it checked out, I called my primary care doctor and described substernal chest pain—a classic symptom of a heart attack. The pain felt like an elephant was sitting on my chest, and I could not expand my chest wall to take in a deep breath. It was the worst pain I had ever experienced, and I have experienced a lot of pain in the past. My primary care physician took me seriously and put me through some testing, which all came back normal. I was reminded again that one's mental state—whether positive or negative—could control one's physical state. The chest pain continued for a week and a half until Leo was born. Not surprisingly, when I first held Leo in my arms and took a big breath, the chest pain immediately dissipated!

Twenty Four

Surrogacy Was Just the Beginning; Parenthood Is Lifelong

Mike and I brought Leo home from the hospital the Wednesday before Thanksgiving. I was nervous about driving that day due to the traffic. I had driven us down to Kyle just a few days earlier on Interstate 35. It's a terrible route to take between Kyle and Dallas any day, but taking it on one of the busiest travel days of the year would be particularly scary. The thought of driving on a busy road with precious cargo on board was too intimidating for me, so I had my husband drive us back home. It normally would have taken my husband about three and a half hours to do this drive, but that day, it took him five and a half. We had to stop to change Leo's diaper and have a quick feed; also, the traffic was terrible, and even though Mike would not admit it, he, too, was scared to drive with our precious cargo on board. It was all too surreal.

Uneventfully, we finally arrived home. Leo was not a happy camper that night—perhaps because he had slept the entire drive home and was now ready to interact, or because he was now in a new environment (i.e., his home), or both—and we woke up feeling like zombies on Thanksgiving Day. We had nothing planned for Thanksgiving since we had not known how things would go with the delivery and hospital visit or when we would be discharged. Nor did we have any family in Texas to go to for Thanksgiving. I was so exhausted that a trip to Boston Market would have been enough.

Mike said he was going to get us something to eat. He returned with a turkey and numerous grocery items. That day, Mike made a special Thanksgiving meal all from scratch, complete with turkey and gravy, stuffing, mashed potatoes, zesty cranberry sauce, and the best lemon meringue pie I had ever eaten. As we said grace that evening before our meal, I realized how much I had to be thankful for. The year 2017 had been the hardest year of my life. God had put me through so many tests, and I had shed so many tears. Yet at that Thanksgiving meal, I realized that God had answered all my prayers. It had taken him a long time to answer them; sometimes, I had not been sure whether he even heard them. But I was truly blessed!

Leo was born a few days before my forty-first birthday. I had received many fantastic birthday presents in the past, but this was truly my best birthday gift ever. The gift of motherhood—a gift I had thought was unachievable. However, my happiness was short lived. From day one of his life, Leo had had a lot of tummy pain;

the doctors said that he was adjusting to living outside the womb and to eating. Unfortunately, at one and half weeks old, he started having bloody diarrhea. Being a physician, I was calm and started a differential diagnostic analysis of the possible causes: bleeding from an anal fissure; wiping his butt too aggressively; thin skin prone to bleeding; a gastrointestinal bug; etc. Since he was eating well and looked hydrated, perhaps this was a gastrointestinal bug that would pass. However, the bleeding became worse very quickly. He then had a massive bloody stool; the diaper was practically all blood. This did not look good. We took several pictures and headed to the emergency room at Children's Plano.

In the ER, the staff performed an evaluation. Because they take babies' temperatures rectally, Leo got to experience the rectal thermometer a few times. We then had the doctor do a guaiac test, which evaluates for bleeding. It involves putting a finger in the anus, obtaining a sample, and then placing the sample on a card. A solution is then dropped on the reverse side of the card. A positive guaiac test will light up once the solution is placed. We really did not need a guaiac test, though, since the blood was obvious in Leo's diaper and on the doctor's gloves. The staff poked him several times to start intravenous fluids and to get a blood sample so they could run tests. It was very difficult for me to watch my son go through this at such a tender age. I suddenly remembered the reason I'd chosen not do pediatrics: it was very tough for me to see children sick and suffering. It was even harder seeing my only child go through this.

Testing was suggestive of a severe milk allergy. I thought they were going to admit him since he was so small, but he looked so good that they had us take him home and switch his formula from Enfamil to Nutramigen. We picked up a can from the pharmacy on our drive home and switched over to the new formula for his next feed. His bloody stools continued. We thought maybe it might take time for the Enfamil to clear his system and for him adjust to the Nutramigen, but two days later, Leo looked worse. For each bottle that he fed, he had three bloody stools. Additionally, he now had sunken fontanels, dry mucosae, a sagging scrotal sac, no urinary output for more than twelve hours, and severe lethargy, being almost unresponsive—all signs of critical dehydration. Amid changing his diaper, we noticed water coming out of his anus—another sign that he was harshly dehydrated.

We returned to the Children's Plano ER, which was crowded this time; it took almost three hours before we were seen. It was difficult to sit in a waiting room in the middle of winter where there were ten children coughing and five children vomiting, including the one sitting right next to us. I was incredibly worried that Leo would pick up an infection. Mike asked me whether I wanted to go home and see the pediatrician the next morning, as we already had an appointment with Leo's doctor then. I felt that Leo was too sick and might not be alive in the morning. The staff was overstressed, and it reflected in the way we were treated. We had a very different experience this time than two days previously, when we'd felt satisfaction and trust in the staff. Again, Leo had multiple rectal temperature checks. He was stuck five times before they were able to get blood; even though he was not a hard stick, he was just too dehydrated. They could not place an intravenous port this time. He was still taking oral fluids, at least, so the doctor gave him some Pedialyte.

The results of Leo's blood work demonstrated that he was critically ill, and his blood count indicated that he was now anemic. Two days earlier, his hemoglobin had been 14 g/dL. Hemoglobin is a protein molecule in red blood cells and is an indication of a patient's blood count. The number drops when there is anemia. Now, his hemoglobin was 10 g/dL. In reality, this 10 g/dL was a hemoconcentrated value; his true value was probably less than that. In two days, he had lost a tremendous amount of blood. Newborns have a very low blood volume compared to adults, so this was a massive loss for someone with such a low volume, and he had lost so much in two days just by pooping. By this time, he had had approximately twelve bloody stools daily for six days. In a seven-pound baby who was barely two weeks old, this was very critical.

Our precious son was transported by ambulance to Children's Dallas, where he was admitted to the neonatal intensive care unit

(NICU). This was the longest night of my life. We had arrived at the ER just before 10:00 p.m. and were finally admitted just after 8:00 a.m. the next day. Once Leo was settled in, Mike and I returned home. We had not slept and felt like zombies. I thought I would be able to sleep now that I knew Leo was safe in the NICU under good care, but I could not. I cried uncontrollably. These were not joyful tears like the ones I had shed two weeks earlier. I knew that if we had not gone to the ER the previous night, I probably would not have had a son that day. In two weeks, Leo had become my everything; I could not imagine a world without him. When I was five years old, I lost my sister Nikki to infectious diarrhea and dehydration. I could not lose another loved one. How had I made it this far in life without someone as precious as Leo?

Twenty Five

The Journey

Leo stayed in the NICU for three days. Upon admission, they switched his formula to Neocate. His bloody diarrhea resolved within a few hours of the switch, and he regained his birth weight by his third day in the NICU. I brought him home on a Thursday. That following Sunday, I was scheduled to run a half marathon in Dallas. Running was a stress reliever for me; I was in a women's running club and had registered for the race many months prior. Several women were running the full marathon and others the half. Although I had started seriously running around age twenty-four, I had never run any official races. I had been good about training for many months, but I had not trained at all during the previous six weeks due to all the circumstances regarding the pregnancy, the delivery, Leo's illness, and a less-than-optimal right knee.

During my training, I developed severe right-sided iliotibial band syndrome (IT band syndrome). I had knee pain from extremely tight muscles, so I stopped running and did a lot of intense yoga during those six weeks. The yoga provided excellent muscle stretching and cardio endurance and was also an outlet for stress. Even though I decided to still run the half marathon, I did not want to run alongside my running partners because I felt guilty holding them back after they had trained so well.

On the morning of the race, Mike and I woke up at 5:00 a.m. to get to Downtown Dallas before the roads closed. I apologized profusely to my husband on the drive there; I was so sorry for making him come out with me, for leaving our son with my recently sick father-in-law, and for the entire year being my fault. Luckily, we left home early that morning, because traffic was terrible. Finding parking was worse. We found a pay-for-parking lot not too far from the convention center. After we parked and paid the meter, we returned to our car and put the ticket on the front dashboard. It was a cold December morning; therefore, I was wearing many layers. I was grateful that my husband was at the start line so I could give him my top layer of clothing. After that, I sent him back home.

I had my phone, identification, credit cards, and cash so I could get a ride home after the race. With another layer of clothes wrapped around my waist, I ran for about seven miles. At mile seven, I heard my husband's voice calling out my name. I was upset with him for not going home yet incredibly happy to see him. It gave me enough mental and physical energy to continue the run. Mike had called home and learned that Leo was doing well with my father-in-law, so he'd stayed for the race, taking another layer of clothes from me now.

The first seven miles were easy. I introduced some walking between miles seven and ten, and I did more walking between miles ten and twelve, but I wanted to run mile thirteen so that I would cross the finish line running rather than walking. Every time I got winded and felt like quitting, I thought about how courageous my son had been just a few days before and how supportive my husband was. They were my inspiration to keep going. I finished the half marathon in an unbelievable two and a half hours. I crossed the finish line running strong, and it was such a good feeling to hear them announce my name. I felt all the pain and stress from the past year melt away. My legs, however, felt like deadweight, barely able to hold me up. Yet I was still able to walk back to the car since the endorphin high made me forget how tired my legs were. The good news was that I did not have any knee pain. The next several days would be spent resting and taking care of my newborn.

After the race, we made it back to Mike's car. Once a woman and her daughter saw me get into the car, however, they pulled my husband aside. About ten minutes earlier, they had seen a woman who was parking next to us bang our car. The saddest thing was that the woman had stayed in that spot next to ours but hadn't left a note under our windshield wipers. Both Mike and I were raised to always do the right thing, even if that thing hurts. Unfortunately, it took many months to fight this, since the woman denied the accident despite photos and eyewitnesses. On the drive home from the race, I again apologized copiously to Mike. If I had not signed up to run the half marathon four months before, we could have been home with our child, who had recently come home from the NICU, and Mike's car would not have damages. I felt so bad; the guilt that everything was my fault diminished the elation of finishing the race.

Granny always told me that nothing in life is easy; life only gets easy after it's over. I will be the first person to tell you that I work exceptionally hard at everything in my life. To the rest of the world, it might seem that I live a perfect life; to me, it has been hard work, with lots of ups and downs. Mike and I got married at an older age. One of the disadvantages of that was that having children was extraordinarily difficult. We work hard at our marriage and our new family, and we discuss everything. I guess Granny was right: life is not easy.

Having a baby has been many years in the making. I had many days of excitement and many more days of pain. We are now parents. Our route to becoming parents was not conventional, nor anything close to conventional. But in the twenty-first century in the United States of America, we have many options to help us achieve parenthood—options that were not available decades ago. Nor are these options available today in certain parts of the world. The journey might not be easy, and there might be detours along the way. But parenthood is a real possibility!

Acknowledgments

First and foremost, I thank God for giving me health and strength for my achievements. He is the reason I am successful today.

I want to thank my patients for their encouragement. I am generally a very private person; many of my friends and family did not know the details of my fertility treatments and surrogacy. As the delivery of my son approached, I started to tell my patients. They were the ones who encouraged me to make my story public. They were the ones who told me that my inspirational story gave them hope and encouragement. Every day, I am forever grateful to my patients for keeping me humble.

Mike, my husband and best friend: thank you for your love and support. Mike was the first person to read this manuscript. I am grateful for your kindness.

Leo, my sweet son: thank you for giving me breaks in between feedings and diaper changes so that I could write this document. You bring more joy to me than I will ever be able to put into words. Your smile and laugh make my heart sweeter than melted chocolates.

Mom and Dad: love and thanks for all the sacrifices you made so I could do something with my life. I know your lives were not always easy, but thank you for your perseverance.

My nephews: thank you for inspiring me every day to have a baby. Spending time with both of you brought me so much happiness that I needed a baby of my own.

Granny: thank you for making me the woman I am today. You have left the biggest mark on my heart. You are my role model and inspiration.

About the Author

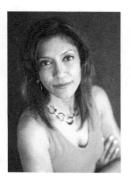 Dr. Dorette Noorhasan is board certified in reproductive endocrinology and infertility as well as in obstetrics and gynecology. After obtaining her doctorate in medicine at Boston University School of Medicine, she completed her obstetrics and gynecology residency through the University of Texas at Houston's Lyndon B. Johnson General Hospital program and her reproductive endocrinology and infertility fellowship at New Jersey Medical School. She is a member of the American Society for Reproductive Medicine, the American College of Obstetrics and Gynecology, the Society for Reproductive Endocrinology and Infertility, and the Texas Medical Association. Dr. Noorhasan has published in numerous journals, including *Fertility and Sterility, Human Reproduction, Women's Health Issues,* the *Journal of Pediatrics,* and *Obstetrics and Gynecology International.*

In this autobiography, Dr. Noorhasan walks you through her personal struggles with fertility and surrogacy and gives a candid description of her life. She is part of an immigrant family who came to America to live the American dream. Through perseverance and hard work, she became a successful fertility physician who has helped thousands of women achieve pregnancy. This book discusses many of the difficult fertility topics that are often ignored and explains what it is like to walk in a patient's shoes.